The Hot Mom to Be
HANDBOOK

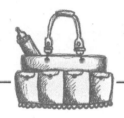

Don't miss the next book by your favorite author.
Sign up now for AuthorTracker by visiting
www.AuthorTracker.com.

The Hot Mom to Be
HANDBOOK

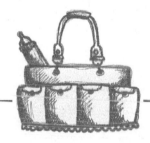

JESSICA DENAY

AVON

An Imprint of HarperCollins*Publishers*

Maternity fashion advice from Rebecca Matthias, president and chief creative officer of Mothers Work, Inc., with brands A Pea in the Pod®, Mimi Maternity®, Motherhood® Maternity, and Destination Maternity®.

THE HOT MOM TO BE HANDBOOK. Copyright © 2010 by Jessica Denay. All rights reserved. Printed in the United States of America. No part of this book may be used or reproduced in any manner whatsoever without written permission except in the case of brief quotations embodied in critical articles and reviews. For information address HarperCollins Publishers, 10 East 53rd Street, New York, NY 10022.

HarperCollins books may be purchased for educational, business, or sales promotional use. For information please write: Special Markets Department, HarperCollins Publishers, 10 East 53rd Street, New York, NY 10022.

First Avon paperback edition published 2010.

Designed by Diahann Sturge

Library of Congress Cataloging-in-Publication Data
    Denay, Jessica.
        The hot mom to be handbook / by Jessica Denay. — 1st ed.
            p. cm.
        ISBN 978-0-06-178735-5 (pbk.)
        1. Pregnant women—Life skills guides.   2. Pregnant women—Sexual behavior.
        3. Mothers—Psychology.   I. Title.
    HQ759.D45   2010
    646.70085'2—dc22

                                                    2009036502

10   11   12   13   14   OV/RRD   10   9   8   7   6   5   4   3   2   1

This Book belongs to Hot Mom *To Be*:

_____

For my son, Gabriel.
You have made my life an adventure.
Thank you for letting me experience the world
through your eyes and heart.

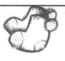

Contents

Big Fat o' Disclaimer

I have been called a mom lifestyle expert, but let me make it clear that I am *not* an expert at being a mom. No one is, or can be: it doesn't matter if you have ten kids or have been parenting for 50+ years, we are all learning day by day, and each child is different, each circumstance is different. Like you, I am doing the best I can every day, making choices, some good ones, some I wish I could do over. Parenting is filled with mistakes; it's about learning from ourselves and learning from others who have been through similar circumstances.

No one is perfect. That is not what this book is about. It's not going to groom you to be the "perfect" Stepford mom, and it's not going to scare you silly with all the potential medical things that could happen. It gives you straight-up, simple, and practical advice, and it's filled with tons of great products to make your pre and post baby life easier and more fun.

Everything has been sourced for you. I should note that the products I recommend were Hot Moms Club tested and approved—none of the companies paid to be included in this book. I chose them solely because the Hot Moms Club team and I tried hundreds of products throughout the years and are privy to the latest and newest on the market. I am sharing our favorites with you.

I am also NOT a doctor, nor do I play one on TV. Always, always, always check with your physician before doing anything new. This book is a guideline and full of great suggestions, but it should never take the place of your doctor's advice. OK, now that we have gotten that cleared up, onto the book. . . .

Preface

I've always said motherhood is about finding a balance,
not balancing everything.

—Gabrielle Reese, professional volleyball player,
Nike spokesperson, fitness expert

A Hot Mom is a woman who is confident and empowered. It doesn't matter what age you are, what shape or size; EVERY mom can be a Hot Mom! It's a choice. It's an attitude and a way of being. It's knowing that you are not the best mom unless you are the best YOU.

You've seen the pink line and now your world is about to change forever. It's already started subconsciously, every time you worry about your baby or change your life to improve hers or his. Motherhood means always anticipating your baby's needs, whether your "baby" is three months or thirty years old. It's aching when your child hurts, and being filled with exuberance at his or her slightest joy.

But motherhood doesn't and shouldn't mean giving up your sense of self. The better you know yourself, the better parent you will be. Your confidence and happiness will be reflected in your children. You are their role model starting day uno, in utero, from the very first moment you become a Hot-Mom-to-be.

I wish I could say this book is a compilation of all the things I did when I was pregnant. But in fact this book is what I learned from my pregnancy and from the thousands of extraordinary mothers I have come to know through the Hot Moms Club (www.hotmomsclub.com) every year. If you're pregnant—or trying—and you don't know what the Hot Moms Club is yet, it's high time you do! We are an online community and emotional and informational resource dedicated to bringing together mothers who refuse to fall into the stereotype of the typical American "mom" category. We're undaunted professionals who are unapologetically sexy or simply dynamic. We break the mold, and we empower each other to redefine motherhood.

The Hot Mom to Be Handbook is filled with things I sure as heck wish I'd known when I was pregnant, as well as advice you better believe I will follow should I ever become pregnant again. It's packed with words of wisdom from experts, thought leaders, and Hot Moms Club members, as well as my crazy friends and relatives. It's real, it's irreverent, but mostly it's inside tips and how-tos from women who have walked the walk (and later waddled the waddle), from the first trimester to the first set of contractions and beyond.

I've made mistakes as a parent, and luckily you will be able to learn from them. I can't turn back time; all I can do is use what I learn to be the best mom I can be today, tomorrow, and the days that follow. Some days I get an A and, well, others . . . let's just say it's not always easy to bridge the gap between knowing things and applying them. But being a Hot Mom is not about being perfect or doing it all. That would be impossible—not to mention boring. Being a Hot Mom is finding balance and happiness in your life so that your child will have a chance at balance and happiness in hers or his. It's about doing your best in each moment and, most importantly, having fun and enjoying the ride, starting right now.

The moment a child is born, the mother is also born. She never existed before. The woman existed, but the mother, never. A mother is something absolutely new.

—Rajneesh

Foreword

My lifelong dream has always been to be a mother. I met my husband, Ryan, on the ABC show *The Bachelorette* (I know . . . crazy!) and became his wife in December 2003. We decided to enjoy our marriage without children for a while. After about a year and a half, we were ready to create a life out of our love and start a family. We tried and tried. Nothing worked. I went to acupuncture, and he had his swimmers checked. We consulted doctors and followed old wives' tales (by the way, standing on your head doesn't work!).

Almost two years later, we found ourselves questioning whether it would ever happen. Before actually "trying," it had never crossed our minds that it would take so long. We thought, *When you have everything in place and want nothing more, isn't it just supposed to happen naturally?* Even though we stayed hopeful and optimistic, it couldn't help but be a downer, especially when my fairy tale wouldn't be complete without a little baby Sutter. After much praying, crying, stress and worry, we were blessed with an EPT test that FI-NALLY read *pregnant*. It was the best shock of my life, and I let out the ugliest happy cry. I would soon learn that the hard part was not over but only beginning, as carrying the baby during pregnancy would prove to take its toll on my body. For sixteen excruciatingly long weeks, nausea ruled my life, and I felt more like a blob than a glamorous pregnant woman. The only things that worked for me, if ever so briefly, were ginger ale, saltine crackers, French fries, Preggie Pops, Fruit Loops, and playing video games (it keeps your mind off your yuckiness!). Living at 8,500 feet elevation, dehydration set in, and one night I blacked out face flat on the bathroom floor. Luckily my husband was home and not on twenty-four-hour fire duty! If that wasn't enough, I got diagnosed with gestational diabetes and had to say good-bye to the pregnancy rite I was looking forward to—stuffing your face with whatever you craved and not worrying about the sugar and caloric consequences! Last, but certainly not least, I ended up developing preeclampsia and HELLP syndrome. I started experiencing nausea and then intense upper abdominal pain; Ryan drove me to the hospital the day before I hit thirty-six weeks. After lots of blood tests and constant fetal monitoring, I progressed to a point that required them to induce. That didn't work as quickly as they needed it to, so they wheeled me in for an emergency C-section, with Ryan in scrubs, holding my hand. After the epidural didn't work, the team of doctors in the operating room jointly decide to put me under general anesthesia. Although it was all hurried and frightening, I woke up three hours later and was introduced to a healthy baby boy who captured me in his sight and didn't let go. Bottom line . . . it was all terrifying, but the light at the end of the tunnel was brighter than anything I could've imagined. Despite the drama we had conceiving and the difficulties of my pregnancy, we wanted another child, and I was willing to go through it all again.

When I married Ryan, I knew without a doubt that I would love him forever and no one would be able to change that. What I didn't think was possible, until we conceived and began to raise a child together, was that the love I had for him would become even deeper and stronger than the day we said "I do." Creating a life out of the love we share created a bond like nothing else. I watch Ryan flying Max around the room or having a conversation through my belly with our unborn daughter, and I fall in love all over again. As a child of divorce, I pray that I will be able to show my kids just how much love and respect I have for their father, because I truly believe that since we are their primary role models, this will help them find long-lasting relationships in the future. They also need to know that their family was started from a place of love and they are a beautiful continuation of that, no matter where we all find ourselves in life.

In anticipation of the birth of my second child, I find myself torn between the excitement of meeting my baby girl for the first time and the utter nervousness of all that comes with her arrival. The fact that the delivery of my firstborn was dramatic and grueling doesn't necessarily give me solace . . . I know what to expect, and my doctors are fully prepared to prevent the rare and terrible medical problems I experienced before, but the worries of a mother still creep in and play with my already weak brain matter. Even more so than my health, I worry about the health of my unborn child. With a son who is now twenty months old and the whispers of my own mother in my ear, I unfortunately know that the worrying will never stop. My biggest worry by far is being the BEST mommy I can be for my two little blessings. And that means being, or at least trying to be, a better version of myself. Imagining that every day is New Year's and the resolutions I usually set and forget about soon after are incorporated into my everyday life. I want my children to learn how to be good people through the examples my husband and I set (not that it's hard for him!). Not only do we have to verbally explain virtues and integrity but we also need to show them, through our own actions, thoughtfulness and loyalty, kindness and consideration, generosity and patience, love, gratefulness, and respect.

Since this is the Hot Moms Handbook, I have to mention that I can't imagine being the best I can be at anything without my health. With my first pregnancy I gained thirty-five pounds, but with baby #2, it's more like an additional fifty. It's not that I worry I can't get back into tip-top shape, I just need to find time and make it a priority. I want to be able to run alongside my son as he rides his bike up and down our little neighborhood in the mountains or go hiking as a family with a fifteen-pound baby on my back. As a realist and a second-time mom, I know that I am low man on the totem pole in our household. However, I plan on taking care of myself not just to look "hot" (although feeling sexy for my husband will be high up on the list too) but also to show my kids the importance of health and wellbeing. I also want to be around for them for years and years and years to come as their "worrying," doting mom, *whether they like it or not!*

—**Trista Sutter, mom of Max and Blakesley**

Special Sections You'll Find Throughout This Book

BUMP ON A BUDGET

Everyone today is looking for ways to save money. For this reason I've included Bump on a Budget, practical tips and ideas in each section to help you tighten your belt as your waistline expands, so to speak. The Discount Guide at the end of the book offers thousands of dollars of savings from some of my favorite preggo retailers.

ECO-MINDED MAMA

It is never too early to start your little ones off to be environmentally conscious and healthy. Thankfully there are many great "green" child-rearing options today from maternity and beyond. In each chapter of the book I have added eco-friendly or organic alternatives to minimize your baby's carbon "butt" print and for your peace of mind.

DADS ARE THE NEW MOM

Dads are more involved than ever in raising children, and it is more socially accepted and expected today than ever before in history. Throughout the pages I share some creative ways to trick—I mean, *get*—Dad engaged and involved in the process even *before* the baby is born.

$TUFF TO DROOL OVER!

The number of luxury baby items on the market (AKA: outrageously priced, and completely overindulgent and unnecessary in every way, yet fabulous) never ceases to amaze me. Just for fun, I have included some of my favorites in various categories sprinkled throughout the book. And for those who are lucky enough to afford them, I provide all of the purchasing information.

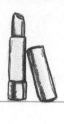

One

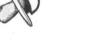

Oh, Oh Baby!

*Making the decision to have a child—it's momentous.
It is to decide forever to have your heart
go walking around outside your body.*

—Elizabeth Stone

The Pink Line

You've got a bun in the oven; you're with child, preggers, expecting; the test is positive—yup, YOU ARE PREGNANT! Whether you had stick in hand and were ready to pee on Day Fifteen, or whether you groggily realized that Ms. Monthly was suspiciously late, for every newly pregnant woman there is that special moment when the full significance of the phrase *I'm going to have a baby!* sinks in. For some, *baby* means excitement, for others overwhelming relief—and still, for others, *baby* means surprise, worry, and disbelief. For me, it was a combination of all of the above. The inner dialogue in my head jumped from *Oh my God, I'm having a baby* to *OH MY GOD, I AM HAVING A BABY!!!???!!!* to *Ooh,*

I'll get to shop for little blue hoodies at Baby Gap to *Ooh, sleepless nights and poopy diapers.* Between thoughts of *Am I ready for this?* and *I'm going to be the best mom ever!* I contemplated whether the babe-to-be would get my smile and his dad's eyes, or his dad's ears and my feet—or, heaven forbid, if my grandfather's nose would suddenly reappear in the gene pool. To top it off, I'd think, *OH MY GOD, my dad is going to know I've had sex!!!* Funny how the mind works and how it can jump from joy to fear to insanity and back again in an instant.

If you've been planning and hoping to get pregnant—if this baby is the exclamation point of a great love—you are truly blessed. Let that gratitude carry you through bouts of morning sickness and the physical difficulties that pregnancy may bring. Fully realize how lucky you are to experience the miracle of life surrounded by absolute joy and anticipation.

> "I've got seven kids. The three words you hear most around my house are 'hello,' 'good-bye,' and 'I'm pregnant.'"
> —Dean Martin

If you are in the surprise pregnancy club (and you're far from alone—about one-third of all births are from unplanned conceptions!), then take a moment to realize that life happens in astonishing and unexpected ways. It's natural to feel a little scared and uncertain. I know I did. I was terrified, yet excited at the same time. I was lucky I had great family and friends to support me and a partner who wanted to be a dad more than anything else in the world. And although things didn't fall into the perfect "plan" that I had for myself or my life, they worked out exactly as they should have, and now, ten years later, I still wouldn't change a thing: my son is and will always be my proudest accomplishment and source of joy. I wish I had realized or known that at the time. Just because you aren't monogramming pillows at week five doesn't mean you're doomed to be a bad mom or that you can't nurture a healthy pregnancy and deliver a thriving baby. Everyone reacts differently. Emotionally and physiologically it is a lot for you to absorb, and it may take you a little time to get in the groove and really feel the excitement. If that is the case for you, know you are not alone and it's OK.

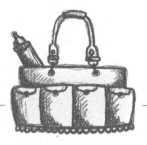

I'm Living My Life Backward

It was a beautiful, warm, sunny afternoon that I'll never forget. The test turned positive in what seemed like less time than one of my heartbeats; as I placed it on the sink, I could already read the result. It made me feel excitement and absolute dread at the same moment.

To say the least, I wasn't prepared for it. At that time in my life I was a senior in college, single, not earning very much money, and not particularly mature. I recognized one solitary factor that eclipsed all else. I was, in fact, pregnant after being told by doctors I would not be able to conceive. There was never even a second of doubt for me. This was my one shot at becoming a mom, and I wasn't going to jeopardize it for anything.

I wasn't even twenty years old, yet on that day I realized that it was the beginning of my son's life. It was also the day my own childhood abruptly ended. I spent my twenties working and being a single mom. In my late thirties, I married and finally got to go away on a honeymoon—and right around the same time my son was preparing to go away to college. In my forties, I went back to school and finished the degree that was interrupted by my unexpected pregnancy. If I continue traveling on this same time line, I'll most likely end up at a sleepover camp in my fifties.

If I had my life to live over, I would change nothing. My son did turn out to be my only biological child and a blessing. He made me into a mom, and without him I would never have felt the gift of love that only exists between a mother and child.

—Elyse Wilk, Hot Moms Club member

BIRTH FACTS

✿ In 1970, the average age for giving birth was twenty-one. In 2000, it was twenty-five. And in 2007, it has risen to twenty-eight. Birthrates for "midlife moms"—women aged thirty-five to thirty-nine—is higher than ever and continues to grow.

✿ The number of moms giving birth in their forties has doubled since 1990.

✿ Of all babies born in the United States each year, 36 percent are born to unwed mothers (roughly 1.5 million).

✿ The oldest woman to give birth was seventy years old.

Don't Worry,
Your Life Won't Change a Bit—Right!

For me, motherhood came much sooner than expected. I was twenty-four, young by today's standards, but not for my mother's generation. Like many women today, I had plans of hitting the snooze button on my biological clock for a while to travel and advance my career . . . yup, that was the plan. Once I found out I was pregnant, I struggled with the reality that my life was about to change forever, as much as I tried to convince myself that it wouldn't.

Not only does your daily routine take a few turns and twists but you as a person have to evolve to rise to the occasion. So if you are still under the delusion that your life is not really going to change that much, it is best you take that notion, crumple it in a ball, and toss it out the window right here and now so you won't be in for a shock. Your life is about to do a 180. It will change in every way you think it might and in ways you never imagined.

"I look at her carefully manicured nails and stylish suit and think she should know that no matter how sophisticated she is, becoming a mother will reduce her to the primal level. That a slightly urgent call of 'Mom!' will cause her to drop her best crystal without a moment's hesitation . . ."

—Dale Hanson Bourke in
*Chicken Soup for
the Women's Soul*

You will soon be able to name all of the SpongeBob SquarePants characters faster than the members of the newest rock band. You'll soon be an expert on every species of dinosaur that ever stomped across the earth and every fairy-tale princess who ever waltzed her way to a happy ending. But the good news—your heart will soon open as big as the universe, wider and more full of joy than you ever thought possible. You will be changed forever, able to love that much stronger in every area of your life. Things that were important to you before will pale in comparison to your child's needs and desires. Yes, your life will be dramatically different, and it will take some adjusting, but you will love it and rise to the challenge. You will find yourself having full-on conversations about the color of your child's poop and, what's more, you'll be excited about it. And, like most parents I know, you will utter the words, "I don't know what I did before my children. I can't imagine my life without them."

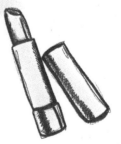

Before and After Kids

Before Kids: You spend your time engaged in intellectually stimulating conversations with your colleagues.

After Kids: Conversation? What's that? Nowadays, you spend your time trying to persuade your child to stop picking his nose in public.

Before Kids: You slip lipstick and a credit card into a sleek handbag on your way out to the mall.

After Kids: You stuff diapers, wipes, animal crackers, sippy cups, Band-Aids, coloring books, crayons, Thomas the Tank Engine, and a bottle of aspirin into your diaper bag on your way out to the playground.

Before Kids: The kitchen floor is so clean you can eat off it.

After Kids: You can eat off the kitchen floor because there's food all over it.

Before Kids: You and your husband consistently enjoy hot sex.

After Kids: You and your husband occasionally enjoy a hot meal.

Before Kids: You coordinate the perfect outfit to wear for a night out dancing.

After Kids: You grab something out of the laundry basket and pray that no one at the puppet show will notice the breast milk stain.

Before Kids: You save money to treat yourself to a Kate Spade handbag.

After Kids: You save money to treat your son to a SpongeBob backpack.

Before Kids: You dine on low-calorie, low-fat lunches at trendy new restaurants.

After Kids: You wolf down someone's leftover pizza and cake at Chuck E. Cheese's.

Before Kids: You can easily finish a great book.

After Kids: You're barely able to finish a simple thought.

Before Kids: Your idea of bliss is being with the love of your life.

After Kids: Your idea of bliss is tucking the love (or loves) of your life into bed each night.

—Comedian Stephanie Blum, mom of three and Hot Moms Club member

Hello Baby: Good-bye Friends?

You may not believe it now, but just as your lifestyle is in for a major "readjustment," your relationship with your friends who don't yet have children is about to change as well. It won't be long before your friends start to think that *you* are preoccupied and boring, fulfilled purely by the musings of your offspring and blinded by their imperfections. And guess what, they will be RIGHT. You may feel that *they* are thoughtless, self-indulgent, or immature and have no idea what it is like to be up every hour with a newborn. And you will be RIGHT. There will inevitably be a shift in your life-style, and although there will be a divide in your respective priorities, there does not have to be a divide in the friendship—just a tweak in its dynamic—as long as you acknowledge and plan. You will have to renegotiate a little bit. Until they have kids of their own, your friends who don't have children may never fully understand the trouble you went to just to show up (late), or the fact that you have to leave early (again) to relieve the babysitter. When the relationship becomes unbalanced and one person feels they are putting in more effort, that's when tension arises. Try to involve your friends as much as possible in your new life as a mom and new baby, but also make time, even if it is once a week or twice a month, for coffee with girlfriends and talk about music, movies, politics, shopping, relationships . . . anything that interested you BC (before child). This will not only please your friends but also help you feel connected and balanced as well.

DADS ARE THE NEW MOM

Remember that your hubby is going through the same adjustment with his friends. If he is the first of his buddies to have children, this can put a lot of strain and stress on him. It is safe to say that his buddies will be less understanding than yours. Women are generally better at making new friends and adjusting to change in their social circles and in life in general. So as the superior species, try to be compassionate to his plight. Be sure, however, to set up some guidelines that will help him carve out time for his friends while still giving you the attention you need and deserve. This might be the perfect time to start befriending other cool couples who either have kids or a baby on the way.

How to Balance Baby and BFFs

Few single experiences can change a woman's life more than having a baby. And as much as our grandmothers, society, our mothers, and other mothers can try and prepare us for the many areas where our lives will morph into something completely different, all due to the sweet little bundle of joy, there is little mentioned or written about the impact this experience can have on our friendships. See, the girlfriend thing remains steadfast and impervious through everything . . . or so they say. The truth is, however, that when a BFF hasn't shared this eternal life-altering experience, there can be tumult, difficulty, tension, and the kind of emotional strain that presents an enormous struggle.

The simple idea that we are not armed, prepared, or even aware that we might be heading into trouble with a friend who doesn't have children is the beginning of what can be something very challenging. As a gender we don't like surprises, especially when it comes to our friends. So the first piece of concrete advice would be to remember to add friendship adjustments to the long list of changes to prepare yourself for when entering the land of motherhood. Note somewhere in your mind that your friendship will require a different kind of attention.

For two women who have had years of

friendship without the responsibility of motherhood, the basic adjustment is a big one when one of them has a child. It affects everything from not having the time to talk on the phone to the little details of everyday life. My best friend in the whole world had her children later in life; she is presently the mother of two kids under the age of three. She came to my house recently, sobbing. When I asked what was the matter, she said, through her tears, "I am so so so sorry, sorry I didn't help you more when your kids were little. I mean I had no idea how hard it was, and now I feel terrible." There it is: we can't expect a friend who has not had a child to be able to understand the transition. And we shouldn't, so keep your expectations low in that area.

There is definitely a give-and-take that can happen. You might figure out ways to incorporate your friend into your new life, such as asking her to be godmother and filling her in on the things neither of you had ever imagined would come up. At a certain point it will become clear that the kind of time you two had in previous days is just not there. Making a standing date such as coffee every Tuesday, or a walk with the stroller every Thursday if you have to bring the baby, is effort that will go a long way.

It's never a bad thing for a mother to remember that for those who don't have children, there might be only so much they can take on the topic. Remember to think and talk about . . . let's say . . . being a woman, or just general life topics. Friends need to be reminded of the bond they had with you before, as they acclimate to the new you (who now has a permanent new appendage).

While juggling an absurd amount just to keep the family and yourself healthy and functioning, it might be hard to imagine our friendships "need" also. But the truth is friendship most definitely requires tending, especially during times of change. If suddenly you realize you haven't had a real conversation with a good friend in weeks, figure out a way to make it happen. As new friends who have children begin to organically fall into position with all you have in common, keep the communication up with the old friend, and tell her about the moms you're meeting. Talk about the adjustment, and share the new as you maintain the old.

Women who don't have children handle this dynamic differently. Depending on a friend's overall life and contentment level, this can be really hard or somewhat seamless. Remember to factor in the reality of your friend's circumstances and her desires. Much like brides, new mothers can fall into the trap of "sorry but it's all about me." Don't do it—our friends are our safety net, our soul holders. They are some of our greatest sources of strength and support. Keep a keen eye and have faith that you will navigate through this much like everything else you've weathered together, and come out closer, stronger, and with new and different memories together, memories that both of you will some day covet almost more than anything you have thus far experienced. Children are the true telltale of the passage of time, and motherhood can bring an even deeper sense of honor and regard to one of most coveted relationships we as women know . . . friendship.

> —Liz Pryor, mother of three,
> columnist, and author of
> *What Did I Do Wrong?*
> *When Women Don't Tell Each Other*
> *the Friendship Is Over*
> (Simon & Schuster/Free Press, 2007)

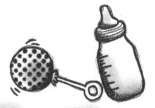

most unbelievable photos and allows you to track every stage of development through extraordinary pictures. If you are already beaming from ear to ear, this book will fascinate you. And if you are having a tough time connecting the knowledge of your pregnancy to the scientific phenomenon going on inside of you, this book will create that synergy.

Use the Force

Amid all the fear and uncertainty during my pregnancy, there was a moment when I really took in what was happening. There was a being, a soul in the making, living inside of me. Let this realization sink in for you. No matter how many emotional hurdles you encounter, marvel in the magic that is growing within you. *Mothers are the most powerful source in the world; we introduce and create life.* From here on, if you choose to, you will be able to tap into the power and strength that only a mother has. There's great wisdom in a mother's instincts. You know, that personal wisdom that allows you to know what's good for you and for your baby. Getting in touch with that instinct is not always automatic for everyone, so slow down for a minute and listen to your inner emotional voice and the rhythm of your body. Recognize your intuition. It's like being a superhero. You've got to trust your powers. As Yoda would say, "You already know that which you need . . . and may the force be with you."

Motherly Instinct vs. Science: Which Force Is Stronger?

I knew I was pregnant even though my blood test came back negative. I told the nurse flat out that the test was WRONG. I felt with conviction that I was with child. I marched right back home and told my husband that the blood test was a "false-negative." He looked at me a bit strangely and even doubted me. He asked, "How can you second-guess the blood test? They are 99.9 percent correct." My answer back was, "Then this is the 0.1 percent chance! Let's wait another week and go back." And sure enough, it happened. Science caught up with my strong motherly instinct! One week later, the blood work came back positive—I was pregnant. And I relished telling both the nurse and my husband, "I TOLD YOU SO!"

—Jennifer Nicole Lee, fitness expert, mom of two, and Hot Moms Club member

Swell . . . And Not Just Your Belly

As your belly starts to expand, let your joy and excitement increase. Attitudes are infectious; the more excited you are about your pregnancy, the more excited others will be about it too. These nine months can lead to better connections with friends and family, a positive transformation of attitude, and an awareness of the possibilities for you and your child. We all have the same innate desire for our babies—we want them to be happy and healthy. And the best way to ensure their happiness is to cultivate your own spirit and enjoyment of life. It is never too early to start.

Start Spreading the News

This is your first opportunity to be not just an ordinary mom but a Hot Mom. Hot Moms take charge of each situation with style and flair, so planning a little fun and excitement in sharing your baby news can start a Hot Mom practice of making events a bit more special. If I could have a "do-over," I would plan a more unique way to tell my son's dad that we were having a baby. He asked me if I was okay because I was acting "strange," and I just blurted out that I was pregnant. No candles, no special dinner, no exciting memory. I can't go back, but I can encourage you—no, urge and beg you—to put some thought into it and share the news in a clever way that reflects the two of you as a couple.

If you opt for a private announcement, maybe you could make reservations at "your restaurant." Dress in your sexy best. Create an evening of romance. Arrange for the waitress to bring a high chair and then spill the news—or simply make the reservation for three! You could stay at home and break out the fancy sparkling water and create a scavenger hunt that leads to a "bun" that you placed in the oven—or some other obvious indicator. You could also choose the old "public declaration"—you know, loudspeakers, intercoms, or a radio station announcing your condition. Whatever way you celebrate the news, make it extraordinary.

Breaking the News

Once you know for sure, it is time to share it with the person you now have by the balls. Here are some creative ways to make it official:

❀ Leave the positive test on the sink and scrawl on the bathroom mirror, Meet me at Babies "R" Us with your wallet and a U-Haul.

❀ Give him a sterling silver rattle with "I think it's yours" engraved on it.

❀ Have the waiter place a personalized message in a fortune cookie: "Confucius says a third of your paycheck is now mine."

—Mary K. Moore, excerpt from
The Unexpected When You're Expecting
(a parody)

I will never forget the day, that amazing moment in time when I found out that my wife and I were going to have a baby. For as long as I can remember, one of my biggest dreams was to be a dad. I am a radio DJ and a bit of a practical joker. When we first started trying, I would often call my wife on air and ask her when she was going to have my baby. We tried for a long time with no luck. Then one day out of the blue, my wife called the studio hotline during my show—something she never did—and told them it was an emergency. I nervously picked up the line, and she said she was pregnant. I thought she was kidding. When I finally realized she was serious, I belted out a huge scream. There are no words to describe how excited and happy I felt at that moment; think a double scoop of vanilla ice cream with all the toppings, *on your day off.* I immediately called my boss, told him I had a "family emergency," then raced right home. And there we were, me, my wife, and "the stick."

— Jack Paper, Radio DJ

This goes for sharing the news with your family and friends as well. If there's a holiday or family gathering in the near future, take advantage of the festivities and add your news to the celebration. Some couples make an emotional toast, but if speeches give you as much anxiety as a root canal, why say anything at all? Dress your three-year-old in an "I'm going to be a big brother!" T-shirt and see how long it takes them to catch on. Or meet everyone at a Chinese restaurant and have fortune cookies made up that say, "You will soon be a grandmother" (or aunt, uncle, etc.) or "I see another baby in your future." At Fancy Fortune Cookies (www.fancyfortunecookies. com), you can customize your message for maximum impact.

At Thanksgiving dinner many, many years ago, my older cousin and her husband stood up to "make an announcement." Everyone thought they were going to tell us that they were pregnant. We all smiled hopefully as images of cooing babies floated in our heads. She excitedly announced that she was off the pill and they were ACTIVELY trying for a baby. She went into a few more details than I choose to remember. In review, telling family and friends at a holiday meal that you are pregnant conjures images of soft little bald baby heads; excitedly telling the group that you are trying like crazy to *make* a baby conjures images of the two of you, well . . . trying to make a baby. That's a Thanksgiving memory no one will thank you for.

Oh Mamma Mia!

The international hit play and movie *Mamma Mia!* centers around a young women determined to have her father at her wedding. The problem, she realizes after reading her mom's diary, is that her father could be one of three men, and the comedy ensues. Now, if you weren't in an exclusive relationship, or if two relationships fell close together, you might not find it so humorous if there are questions about who the father of your baby might be. If you find yourself in this scary and stressful predicament, take a deep breath; fortunately, there are many inexpensive and easy ways to determine paternity today. This may not solve some of the emotional issues you are bound to face, but knowing will help your peace of mind and ability to plan for the future. Doctors generally do not advocate prenatal paternity testing, because the tests are invasive and carry some risk for the fetus. Most physicians will suggest waiting until the baby is born, when paternity testing can be done safely and painlessly.

Paternity, however, *can* be determined through amniocentesis, a genetic testing procedure done between fourteen and twenty-four weeks of pregnancy on women who either have an abnormal ultrasound, a family history of birth defects, or who are thirty-five years or older. This test is used to find certain genetic abnormalities, but paternity and the gender of the baby can also be determined if requested. Amniocentesis is performed by a doctor; a needle is inserted into the uterus to grab fluid from the amniotic sac surrounding the fetus. The fluid is sent to a lab, and results are returned anywhere from a few days to a few weeks. If you are scheduled for amniocentesis, the lab can also run tests for paternity, though there might be some cost involved, depending on what is covered by your insurance.

Now *you* may be certain about the paternity, but people around you may be urging you to get tested. I was in an exclusive relationship with my son's dad when we were surprised by the pregnancy, and unless I was artificially inseminated by some random guy at a bar, there was no doubt in my mind who the father was; he was the only person I had been intimate with in many, many months. However, from the time we announced that we were expecting, his mother insisted and questioned whether the baby was truly his. She strongly urged, and practically begged for, testing. I was naturally hurt and offended by this, so if you are in a similar position, it is understandable to feel insulted. The irony is now that my son is nine and getting older, and if he were to tell me in ten years that a girl he was dating was pregnant, I would want them to take a test as well. It would have nothing to do with the girl, just as my mother-in-law's wishes had nothing to do with me or my character, and just like it has nothing to do with you. Try to remember it is most likely not personal, just a mother being protective of her son—something I can now relate to, and something someday you will be able to relate to.

In case you were wondering, we never ended up taking the test. My ex—my son's dad—never wanted to, although I encouraged it, both for his mom's peace of mind and to affirm what I already knew (I secretly wanted the "I told you so" moment). We never went down that road, though there were many times afterwards when I wish we had, as it would have ended the countless questions from my in-laws and inspections on who he looks like, etc. . . . So if you know, and want others to have that same confidence, there is no harm, aside from your bruised ego, in testing once the baby is born. It's a simple procedure, and painless: DNA samples are gathered via cotton swabs from the mouth of the baby as well as the father and the mother, then sent to a lab to analyze. It usually takes three to five days to get the results, and, depending on where you go, can cost from $89 to $400. There are even some over-the-counter paternity tests, but something as important as this is worth spending a little extra money on. Making sure you are in professional hands means there is less of a risk for error.

For more information, talk to an expert in the field or go to DNA Services of America www.dnasoa.com. They have locations and consultants nationwide that can answer your questions in depth.

Can You Keep a Secret?

If this is a pregnancy that's been a long time in the making, you might be so excited that you tell every-one in your Facebook account in less than four minutes . . . or Twitter the news to the entire planet in a matter of seconds. But sometimes, for any number of reasons (work, family issues, medical conditions), you may not want *everyone you have ever said hello to in your entire life* to know about your "delicate condition." However and whenever you decide to announce your pregnancy, just do what feels right and comfortable for you.

But don't feel bad if you're not successful in keeping it hush-hush until the third month. If you're headed to the bathroom every twenty minutes to throw up, or if your skin is glowing and you've suddenly taken an in-terest in baby strollers, you may not be able to keep your secret for very long. So if there are people you think should hear firsthand (like your boss or your family), tell them sooner rather than later (before that bitch at the reception desk or your sister-in-law "outs" you for hurling in the bathroom). And, of course, once you start communicating the news, it will spread. Gossip is part of human nature, and even your most cautious request about "keeping the secret" will be disregarded by some overly excited recipients of the news. Just what you want—one of your office mates shouting across the cubicles, "Hey, keep it a secret, but I happen to know Jess is packing a baby!" And a good rule of thumb: key into positive energy first! Make plans with that friend or coworker who openly loves being a mom. She will get you psyched up—and good role models and understanding buddies are invaluable during your pregnancy.

> *"You should never say anything to a woman that even remotely suggests that you think she's pregnant unless you can see an actual baby emerging from her at that moment."*
>
> —Dave Barry

Preggo 9 to 5

Now, if you are a Hot Mom, it is most likely that you are a valuable employee. Keep in mind that as friendly as you are with your boss on a personal level, and as excited as your coworkers may genuinely be for you, they still have to fill your position when you're gone, and there will be some natural concern over whether you really will come back after the baby is born. This can be stressful for them, so try to keep that in mind when approaching the situation. Grab them in a good mood or right after you just finished a big project or got praised for a job well done. Be sure you sit down with your boss in a private place, and be confident and excited. You may be nervous inside, but try not to let that show. Reassure your employer that you love working there and how much your job means to you now that you will have to provide for a child. Let them know that you will do whatever it takes to make sure the transition for your replacement is as smooth as possible.

HOW *NOT* AND WHEN *NOT* TO TELL YOUR BOSS YOU ARE PREGNANT

❀ Stop him while he is rushing off to an important meeting

❀ Tell EVERYONE else in the office first and then tell your boss

❀ While she's stressed or on a deadline

❀ While he's hungry and heading to lunch break

❀ During her lunch hour

❀ Before an evaluation

❀ Complain about your morning sickness and sore back and toss in how tired you are

❀ Cry a lot and tell them how emotional and hormonal you are right now

Maternity Leave

Know your rights and your options. Now I am no legal expert, but below is a summary, or the "Cliffs Notes" version, of everything I have researched and read regarding maternity leave. Policies and guidelines vary from state to state and company to company. Before you tell your boss, it is important to know what you can expect in your given field. Research on the web, hit your local library, and talk to your Human Resources Department about your company's specific policies. Ask a colleague you trust who recently had a baby what her experience was like, both logistically and emotionally.

The Law

FMLA (Family and Medical Leave Act) is a federal law that gives both male and female employees twelve weeks of unpaid leave after a birth. It also ensures that when you come back your job will be waiting. Although they aren't required to pay you for this time, your employer must continue your health benefits while you are on leave. You qualify for FMLA if you work for the federal, state, or local government, or for any company with more than fifty employees within seventy-five miles of your workplace. You must have worked for the company for at least a year and at least 1,250 hours during that year. If you and your partner both work for the same company, you receive only twelve weeks combined.

The laws for maternity leave vary from state to state, so make sure you research what additional benefits your state offers. Below I list a few of the states with the most generous laws:

Hawaii: All working women are eligible for maternity leave and may collect 58 percent of their salary from the state for up to twenty-six weeks.

California: Workplace must have at least five employees. California allows pregnant women to collect disability for six to eight weeks after childbirth and collect two-thirds of their salary up to $490 a week.

Rhode Island: All women may qualify for disability for up to 60 percent of their salary, up to $504 dollars a week.

Unbelievably, the United States and Australia are the only industrialized countries that don't provide paid leave for new mothers. France, Poland, Russia, Spain, Austria, Brazil, and Costa Rica are just a few of the many other countries that offer four to six MONTHS' leave after childbirth with 100 percent salary paid. Italy and Sweden give new moms five months' leave and 80 percent of their income.

DADS ARE THE NEW MOM

Paternity leave is becoming more common with men today, but still only about 15 percent of men actually apply. Financially it is not as realistic, and for a long time most men felt a negative cultural stigma, which is now changing. The importance of family bonding is becoming more accepted and smiled upon. Major companies like Ikea, Merrill Lynch, and Microsoft have been known to give paid paternity leave.

Making the $$

Since taking twelve weeks' unpaid leave is not realistic for most couples today, many employers will luckily allow you to use accumulated sick leave, vacation, and personal days so that you can continue to get a paycheck. You can distribute those twelve weeks however you like; you can take them all at once, or break them up and shorten your work week to four days in the child's first year.

Check to see if short-term disability insurance is available as part of your benefits package. It covers your salary or portions of it when you can't work due to injury, illness, or childbirth.

"OUR Baby"

Telling your other baby that there will be a new member in the family can be tricky, depending on your child's personality and age. It's important to develop excitement; remember, they are used to being the center of your world, and sharing you will be harder than sharing their favorite toys.

When I was at the park with some friends and their kids, I asked the young ones, "Where do babies come from?"

Cooper responded, "Under Mommy's shirt."

"The stroller," Sarah said.

"No," Alana put in, "babies come from *the hospital*."

Children under the age of two will understand once you actually start showing, but children older than four are capable of understanding that a new baby is on the way whether they can see a bump or not. Experts suggest that you start telling them as soon as you start telling everyone else. This is a great opportunity to teach your other child/ children about the process. You can show them picture books and discuss the stages as your tummy expands. Relate everything back to when *they* were in your tummy. Stories about the stork may seem cute, but they will make it more difficult for your little one to really understand. Refer to the baby as *"your* baby" or *"our* baby" instead of *"my* baby" or *"the* baby." Let siblings help pick out clothes and toys for "their" baby and ask their advice for decorating the nursery. If you encourage them any way you can and help foster a connection for them, this will help lessen jealousy later on. Just a reminder: kids are capable of understanding, but very few are capable of keeping secrets, so if you tell your oldest or your niece or nephew or that cute little neighbor boy next door, rest assured that they will be so excited that they'll tell their teacher at school and anyone within earshot. Telling them *not* to tell is like trying to fight a fire with a water gun . . . pointless.

If you have a blended family or stepchildren, this can be a bonding experience for the whole family—the glue and blood that connect you all—when presented correctly. Make sure the other child or children feel how excited you are that they will be part of the process and just what an important job being a big brother or sister is. One of the biggest fears children have is that you will love the baby more than them or feel that you don't need them anymore. Making sure they understand their place and worth in the family will only make the experience smoother for everyone.

Big Babies

Use the techniques above with your hubby as well, as he is, in fact, your first baby or "big baby." If you're having your first child, up til now your husband has been used to your undivided attention. He truly feels he is the center of your universe. Praise him for the great father you know he is going to be and how devoted he is to taking care of you. A little encouragement goes a long way, and, like all things spoken and thought, it can become a self-fulfilling prophecy.

Men are simple: like dogs and toddlers, they respond to praise and treats. (Oh yeah, and a little heavy petting goes a long way. . . .)

Remember Your Husband Is Pregnant Too
(Minus All of the Hard Stuff)

Most moms I know are looking for a way to get their husbands more engaged and excited about the baby in the beginning. It's easier for Dad to relate as your tummy grows and after they are given some responsibility, whether it's building the crib, aiding in childbirth, or holding an actual baby. While we women love reading and preparing, most guys I know would rather cut off their arm and eat it than read a long pregnancy book or sit through classes.

So if you want to get your husband prepared—and if you want to earn major brownie points—order a pizza, get him a six-pack of beer, and pop in the DVD *Being Dad* (www.beingdadusa.com). It's a hilarious take on pregnancy from "real" men, it's entertaining and informative, and if you watch it with him it can really open up an honest dialogue of how you both feel about the big changes ahead.

And although he isn't going through morning sickness, exhaustion, or constipation, he is trying to support you emotionally (AKA, deflect, decipher, and tame your mood swings) and sort out his own feelings about everything from your sex life to financial considerations, to his relationships with his buddies, all while dealing with baby-related projects and questions from relatives So again, as the superior species, keep this in mind!

The Other Man . . . or Woman

Not only will you need the support of your friends and family but your doctor (OB) will also be one of the most important people in your life for the next nine months— and she or he will have a great influence on your pregnancy. It is crucial that you seek out a doctor you love and who shares your views of pregnancy and birth. Find a doctor you feel comfortable with and trust implicitly.

It's no secret that pregnant women have tons of questions, and I was on the top end of that scale. (I am sure there were many times I made my doctor regret ever going to med school.) I knew I had struck gold when my OB sat for over an hour and answered all of my many questions, even the ridiculous ones, without a snicker. His all-knowing, "I've-done-this-a-million-times, don't-worry-about-a-thing" smile never left his face.

Not all doctors were created equal, so do your research. You are trusting him or her with your health and the health of your baby; is there anything more important than that? I have heard horror stories, so get referrals from friends. And make sure you *like* your doctor; he or she may have all the degrees in the world, but if your personalities don't mesh, it's better to find someone else, whom you like and trust. Let's face it—this doctor will be with you for some pretty big milestones, from hearing your baby's heartbeat for the first time to the "Big Day."

It is equally important to make sure you and your doctor have the same ideals and birth plan scenarios. Whether you have visions of a home water birth with low lights and soft music, or you plan on taking drugs the second your water breaks, your doctor needs to be aware and on the same page as you are.

GET A HYBRID

Gynecologist: a doctor specializing in female reproductive organs and diseases

Obstetrician: a medical doctor specializing in pregnancy and births

OB-GYN: a physician who specializes in both!

Absolutely No McSteamys or McDreamys Allowed

There should be some sort of rule about doctors being too handsome—it should not be allowed. A friend of mine had a dashing doc and shared her experience: "Before every appointment, I felt like I had to get 'ready.' Truthfully, it was a little much looking down during delivery. It felt a little like having that cute guy on the football team who you would never be able to date deliver your baby. I always felt a little tongue-tied and awkward around him. He was a smart, caring, good doctor, but every visit I felt like an awkward schoolgirl."

The last thing you want to be worrying about is if your doctor will think you are waxed right or if you gained a few extra pounds. Do you really want to talk to him about that hemorrhoid on your butt or how you are gassier than a drunken sailor? No. You may leave out important info because you are too embarrassed to discuss with him some of those, um . . . "perks" of pregnancy. The nice thing is you can let him down easy by saying, "I really like you . . . you seem like a nice doctor, but this is just not going to work for me."

It has also been said that sometimes patients fall for their doctors. When your hormones are going crazy, and you are not thinking straight, and your doctor is extending patience and care and concern, it can often be mistaken for interest. If your doctor looks like Elmer Fudd, this will be less likely to happen to you! So do yourself a favor; if you run into McSteamy or McDreamy on your quest to find the perfect doctor, McRun out of there!

GOING ON A DUE DATE?

Your doctor will give you a due date. In case you can't wait, the traditional way to calculate it is to subtract three months from the last day of your menstrual period and then add seven days. If that proves too confusing, there are due date calculators online. Go to www.marchofdimes.com and search *due date calculator.* But don't rely on the date too much; it's just a point of reference. You can deliver a few weeks before and up to two weeks late.

FACT

Only 5 in 100 moms actually give birth on their due date!

So, Hot Mom, are you ready for the next eight months? Make sure your support team is too, and get rarin' to go for . . . not a bumpy ride but a ride with your bump.

$TUFF TO DROOL OVER

Baby planners, just like wedding planners, are all the rage in Hollywood. With the unbelievable amount of information and products on the market today it is hard to know what is best for your lifestyle. There are many personal services (paid hourly or on a flat consulting fee for personal attention) that will answer all your questions, your late-night phone calls, and your casual concerns. One great resource is Baby Planners (www.thebabyplanners.com). Their motto is "we take the labor out of your delivery." Melissa Gould and Ellie Miller are moms and consultants and are on parent-to-be speed dials everywhere!

BUMP ON A BUDGET

The Hot Moms Club works with high-profile celebrity moms in creating the perfect nursery, baby shower, and sourcing out the best products for their celebu-spawn. Many of the tips and secrets we share with them are in this book and on our website. If you don't have family near and can't afford a personal baby planner, jump on the web and research. www.hotmomsclub.com is a great resource for information and meeting moms in your area. We have groups on Facebook, Twitter, and MySpace, making it easier than ever to meet your cyber soul sister! Plus it's free! We can't stress enough the importance of having a "baby buddy"—someone you can rely on for advice, someone to lean on through the ups and downs and to share the funny moments, as well as the less glorious ones, with.

Two Peas in a Pod—*Literally*

I have never had twins, but several of my good friends have. If you're having twins, it seems you are in good company and, in fact, right on trend these days! Twins are the latest phenomenon/fad to hit Hollywood, or, as some now call it, "Twinseltown." Some of the most famous and most respected actresses have given birth to twins, including Angelina Jolie, Julie Roberts, Jennifer Lopez, Holly Hunter, Geena Davis, Joan Lundon, Nikki Taylor, Jane Seymour, Julie Bowen, Holly Robinson Peete, Marcia Cross, Angelea Bassett, and Rebecca Romijn, to name a few.

The number of twins born since 1980 has risen more than 50 percent, and the number of multiple births (triplets, quadruplets, quintuplets, etc.) has risen more than 400 percent. Assisted reproduction and women having children at older ages, when twinning is more common, may explain the increase.

If you are expecting twins, congratulations. There are so many great resources, support groups, and books available for you on the web and in stores today. I have never had twins, so I can't speak any great words of wisdom; all I can do is point you in the direction of those who can. After consulting with my network of moms who have multiples, these were their favorite go-to spots for information or products.

Resources:

MOST—Mothers of Supertwins (www.mostonline.org)
Twins magazine (www.twinsmagazine.com)

It's Twins! by Susan Heim (www.amazon.com)

Trendy Twin Shop (www.trendytwinshop.com)

Created by identical twins, Just Multiples (www.justmultiples.com) is an online site with all the cutesie twin and multiple products you can handle, from funny onesies with sayings like *I'm the favorite* to triple and quad strollers. For products for multiples, this site is a great reference.

FUN TWIN FACTS

✿ The chances of having fraternal twins naturally is roughly 1 in 300, also fraternal twins run in families.

✿ Triplets occur approximately 1 in every 8,000 naturally conceived births.

✿ The world's first IVF, or "test tube" babies as they were then called, were twins Stephen and Amanda Mays born June 5, 1981.

✿ Multiple births make up only about 3 percent of all deliveries.

✿ Cirque du Soleil employs the most sets of twins.

✿ Once you have had fraternal twins, you are three to four times more likely to have another set!

❀ Identical twins have the same DNA, but not the same fingerprints: no two people have the same fingerprints, not even identical twins.

Blogging the Baby

You are entering one of the most exciting times of your life, so record it in any and every way that you possibly can. You will never regret having those videos, photos, journal pages, or blogs. *Blog* wasn't even a word when I was pregnant, but baby blogging is quite the rage now. So if you're glued to the computer, you might find it more convenient to start a pregnancy blog than a paper journal. It's free, and you can easily update and share your daily experience and photos with family and friends. You can continue to keep the online journal and photos after the baby is born so those out-of-town relatives will be able to track kiddo's progress.

I still prefer the traditional route when it comes to sentiments. There's something about writing in a journal—the scratch of pen on paper—and the fun of putting in other clippings and notes that seems so much more real. I found my pregnancy journal the other day and began reading it. What a treasure it was for me to go back and read the insights of a twenty-four-year-old girl embarking on a whole new chapter in her life. It was thrilling to relive the fear, the joy, and the sheer honesty of it all. Our minds and memories are selective, and this brought back things I had completely forgotten. Regretfully, I didn't keep it up. The journal ended just before the three-month mark. I am devastated that those details, the inner workings of my pregnant mind, are lost forever. If I could go back, I would shake myself and say, *Take the five to ten minutes to write down your thoughts and skip that rerun of* Seinfeld *or* Melrose Place.

I encourage all you Hot Moms-to-be to start today and write everything down; no matter how silly the thought, or crazy or weird, write it down. Write your cravings, what people are telling you, what makes you laugh, what scares you silly—don't miss a thing. You will treasure those pages someday, and I guarantee your little one will too. If I was in search of a baby journal today, I'd visit the Tummy Talk website (www.tummy talk.com) because they have, in my opinion, the most adorable and versatile albums—journal and scrapbooks all in one!

Baby Love Letters

Your lifelong relationship with this little person who calls your tummy home has already started. You're already spending hours thinking about, hoping for, and otherwise imagining who it is you're so close to but can't yet see. Put all these thoughts on paper now—all of your daydreams about your first snuggle with your baby, your child's someday first bike, even what her or his own babies will be like way down the road. . . . I mean, c'mon, nine-plus months is a long time to think; your mind definitely wanders.

Before sleep deprivation robs you of these musings, get them memorialized. Write your unborn pumpkin a love letter. Detail the first kick, the way he seems to bump into your ribs with laserlike aim, the circles she turns like an acrobat, how your heart might have even stopped beating for a smidge the first time you saw him up on the ultrasound screen. This is the stuff you'll want to read about in a month, a year, a decade . . . and that's to say nothing of what your son or daughter will think of this stack of love letters about all the expectations you had when you were expecting.

Canopy Cards (www.canopycards.com) of-fers a package of ten letterpressed note cards so you can write your baby a love letter each time he or she hits a milestone. The cards are packaged beautifully and make a great keep-sake for when your "baby" is all grown.

—Jennifer Parker

Another great keepsake is Anne Geddes's *My Pregnancy Calendar*, which is filled with beautiful photos of babies and pages for re-cording your thoughts and feelings, infor-mation from doctors visits, etc. . . . it's a gorgeous book you'll want to save forever (www.annegeddes.com).

Journal—Month One

If you're like me, you may have trouble getting started with a journal—or keeping one up. So I'm including a few journal questions at the end of every chapter just to get (and keep) the ball rolling.

1.   What were your first words or thoughts when you found out you were pregnant? And be honest!

_____

_____

_____

_____

_____

_____

_____

_____

_____

_____

_____

_____

_____

_____

_____

_____

_____

_____

_____

_____

2. What are you the most excited about? What do you fear the most?

_____

_____

_____

_____

_____

_____

_____

_____

_____

_____

_____

_____

_____

_____

_____

_____

_____

_____

_____

_____

_____

_____

_____

3. What was the funniest thing that someone said or
    did when you told them about "the bun"?

_____

_____

_____

_____

_____

_____

_____

_____

_____

_____

_____

_____

_____

_____

_____

_____

_____

_____

_____

_____

_____

_____

_____

_____

_____

4. Once you're pregnant, you notice every baby in the world. How many babies did you see today?

_____

_____

_____

_____

_____

Two

Womb with a View and a Sound System

It is said that the present is pregnant with the future.

—Voltaire

My son's first words were "Vinny, no!" That's right; not "Mama" or "Duda" but "Vinny, no!" I know you may be thinking, *Who is Vinny? And what does this story have to do with me?* Let me explain. We had two black Labradors, Vinny and Dante, and they both *loved* the baby. Vinny especially. Picture the friendliest, most excitable, playful dog . . . *on caffeine.* That was Vinny. Vinny could hardly contain himself around the baby. Every chance he got, he would lick, sniff, and slobber all over him. From the day we brought our son home, we would remind Vinny, "No licking the baby, Vinny!" and "No, Vinny, step back from the baby!" and "Vinny, no, no, NO!"

All during this time, like every mom, I would gaze into my son's eyes and say "Mama" a hundred or so times a day in hopes he would acknowledge me. "Say 'Mama,' Gabe." Despite all my prodding, one afternoon while I was dressing Gabriel, Vinny came over to give him a wet kiss—and my son's first words were "Vinny, no!" Kids are so perceptive; they are taking in everything, not just what you consciously provide. You never can tell what they are ingesting mentally; it's so important to be aware of what's going on around you, and how your child is responding . . . even in utero!

Paging the Mother Ship

Your child's awareness of her or his environment begins in the womb. That's right, even in your uterus your baby is picking up everything that is happening in your world. You may be playing Mozart an hour or so a day, but if you're having a nightly fight with your husband (or mother-in-law or sister), or if your job has you anxious beyond belief, you might be creating a tense and stressful experience for your little one. They don't pick up only what we direct at them—they are taking in EVERYTHING.

Just as your body and mind work together, you and your unborn baby are functioning as a unit. To me, it's as if you're an ocean ship and the baby is a passenger. (Sail with me on this one!) Imagine your pregnant body as the vessel for a special passenger. Sure, this shapely ship called "mom" is self-contained, darn safe, and built to withstand rough weather—and of course the pilot is skilled at navigating the seas. But no matter how good the piloting, that precious passenger in the hold will experience all the literal and figurative ups and downs of this maiden voyage! Just as on a real ocean trip, changes in air, fuel, temperature, and the mood of the crew will affect the little traveler. I personally would like to sail the metaphoric Bahamas and skip monsoons and the Antarctic chill, but life sometimes gives you rough waters.

From the moment of conception until your nine months are up, your baby is exposed to your database and interpretations of the world—and during this time your baby's brain is forming, memory is beginning to be structured, and emotional patterns are started. That means your thoughts, emotions, and feelings translate into molecules, mainly hormones, which flow into the body of your fetus. Life learning begins BEFORE birth, and experiences before birth can actually affect and mold your baby's personality and nervous system development. In order to give your little one the best beginning, you have to keep yourself in the best frame of mind.

> "Since I became pregnant, my breasts, rear end, and even my feet have grown. Is there anything that gets smaller during pregnancy?"
> "Yes, your bladder."
> –Author unknown

Having a Baby? Adopt a Sense of Humor

One sure way to alleviate stress is to activate your sense of humor . . . about everything. You'll have plenty of time to worry and feel guilty after the baby is born—it comes with the title Mom! Seriously, most things have a humorous side, especially when you realize that almost anything you experience has happened before. Don't they always say that the best humor comes from a bit of misery? Next time morning sickness hits, remember that by the time your baby is born, it will be gone!

Channeling the Zen Mom Inside You

Another great coping strategy is to engage your inner calm. There are any number of ways to physically and mentally bring yourself back to your center. You probably have a few of your own personal favorites. So start putting into practice a regimen of deep breaths and warm baths. If you've ever had a meditative practice, this might be the time to renew it. Take walks, listen to your favorite music, and reassure yourself (and your baby) that everything is all going to be okay. When you are calm and centered, you are providing the ideal situation for your little one to grow.

Just as important as creating a tranquil environment is taking care of yourself physically. Everything in your environment is passed on to your baby—the things you smell, the baby smells; the things you feel, the baby feels; and the things you eat and drink, the baby ingests. If you've spent years thinking about changing your diet or eating healthier, there has never been a better time than now. Start today to consciously move toward taking better care of yourself emotionally and physically. It's an art you can carry with you the rest of your life. What could be more motivating than contributing to the health of your baby?

Water You Talking About?

How many times have you heard "Drink eight glasses of water a day"? I know what you're thinking; you can barely keep track of your car keys, let alone how many glasses of water you drink. But like it or not, hydration has never been more important than now. Did you know that the human body is 75 percent water and 25 percent solid matter and that the brain is almost 85 percent water—and is extremely sensitive to dehydration? Many people think that tea, coffee, and juice count toward the daily water needs of the body. Although these drinks contain water, they also contain dehydrating substances, such as caffeine. These substances rid the body of the water they are dissolved in as well as the body's water reserve. So when you drink coffee or tea, your body expels more water than what is contained in the drink.

From the time of conception until the baby is full-term, just about a trillion cell divisions take place, and these new cells have to be filled with water. It is crucial that you take in more water than ever to keep both you and the baby fully supplied. The water we drink carries nutrients through your blood and to your baby, while your placenta provides around one cup of water necessary every hour to replenish the amniotic fluid in the womb. Moreover, drinking enough water helps prevent urinary tract infections, and, ironically, you are less likely to retain water if you are well hydrated.

If you are like me and forget or find it challenging to drink enough water, you will need to make an extra effort. I came up with a few tricks to help make this easier and tastier. If keeping track of eight glasses seems more challenging than an algebra problem, buy a liter of water and drink two a day; that's much simpler to manage. I would also invest in a clear pitcher that can hold two liters or more. Fill it with water, and—if you want, for fun—drop in thinly sliced lemons, limes, oranges, and cucumbers. Throughout the day, pour yourself water from your pitcher. When the pitcher is empty, you've had the proper amount. If you get bored with plain water, Hint (www.drinkhint.com) has the most delicious naturally flavored water, with no sweeteners or preservatives. The peppermint is outstanding and helps with nausea. Also, adding frozen fruit like kiwi, peach, orange, apricot, and plum instead of ice cubes will make any plain glass of water more fun and refreshing; the frozen fruit looks colorful and cools your drink with a hint of flavoring.

H2 Ought Oh . . .

It is important that you filter your tap water in general, but especially when you are pregnant. There are various types of filtration systems that go right on your faucet, in addition to portable Brita systems, to keep water clean and fresh. This is worth the investment during pregnancy and beyond.

Bottled water is more popular than ever; it is even hard to avoid. Just be aware that many plastic water bottles include bisphenol-A (BPA), a chemical that is potent and mimics the estrogen hormone in the body. Studies have found that freezing, heating, or reusing the plastic water bottles can cause the BPA to leach into your water. Refillable stainless steel bottles are a safe alternative.

ECO-MINDED MAMA
No more plastic bottles! The Intak by Thermos is a BPA-free refillable water bottle. It has a built-in filter, and the cap is numbered and rotates so you can keep track of how much water you are drinking!

BUMP ON A BUDGET
For the amount of water you will be downing, purchasing one reusable thermos or stainless steel water bottle for around ten dollars is cheaper in the long run than buying plastic bottled water. If you have a refillable bottle already, put eight rubber bands around it in the morning and take one off each time you refill it—that's a quick and cheap solution that will help you keep track of the number of glasses you drink during the day!

No Caffeine, No Alcohol, No Smoking, Oh My

Caffeine

Just as water is helpful and goes right to the baby during your pregnancy, caffeine runs through the same pipeline. I am sure your doctor has already told you that caffeine passes through the placenta and into the umbilical cord blood easily, and that developing fetuses sustain higher levels of caffeine than you do because their metabolism is not fully developed. If you are a coffee junkie, now is the time to wean yourself. It may be hard to cut it out completely, but cutting back will benefit you and your baby. Switching to decaffeinated coffee and tea is one way to cut down on your intake while still getting the taste and fix. Keep in mind that decaf coffee still has a few milligrams of caffeine. And a twelve-ounce glass of iced tea or any hot tea that is not decaffeinated generally has almost as much caffeine as a cup of coffee.

Alcohol

I have heard from friends that they feel it is safe to have a glass of red wine now and then during pregnancy. Again, because alcohol passes rapidly through the placenta, no doctor I spoke with recommended drinking ANY form of alcoholic beverage during pregnancy—not hard liquor, not beer, not a mixed drink, wine cooler, or even an occasional glass of wine. The physicians I spoke with agreed that because the fetus cannot break down the alcohol like an adult, it puts them at risk for a variety of birth defects and slows their development. Ask your doctor and follow what he or she suggests. Now, I'm no prude, and I'm generally pretty easygoing, but I am of the opinion that it's better safe than sorry when it comes to the health of the baby.

Smoking

If you are a smoker, STOP. If your partner or relative smokes strongly, encourage them to stop, especially around you! Secondhand smoke is dangerous for your unborn baby. Exposure to the combination of carbon monoxide and nicotine in cigarette smoke can cause serious health problems for your child.

It is said that the sense of smell is the first of the senses to develop in utero. Your unborn baby can take in the environment just as you do, good or bad. As a rule of thumb, any smell that displeases you or feels too strong will most likely be harmful to your fetus. And just as you do your best NOT to inhale cigarette smoke, paint fumes, smog, or harmful chemical smells, try to surround yourself with pleasing smells, even subtle smells like the morning dew, or stronger scents like lavender, cinnamon, lemon, lime, or fresh baked cookies or bread. Anything that makes you smile will have a pleasing effect on your little passenger as well. Smells like curry or spice or anything directly associated with your culture is imprinted in the baby beginning in the womb.

Do Not Stress . . .
<u>I Can't Stress This Enough!</u>

Okay, all you Hot Moms-to-be, I realize that you may be freaking out right now because right before you found out you were pregnant you had one too many glasses of wine at a cousin's engagement party, or because two weeks ago you snuck a smoke with a coworker, or because you had a complete meltdown when they were out of persimmon ice at the gelato shop. Take a deep breath right now! You can't change the past or worry about things you did before you knew. That will just make you more stressed. And, furthermore, occasional difficulties or a stressful day aren't the big worry—really, it's chronic stress that can have long-term effects on you and your baby.

Face it: it is unrealistic to think that our lives will ever be stress-free—or that we will never feel overwhelmed, angry, or frustrated. But acknowledging that we must do our best to control our reactions to difficult people, unplanned events, and life's many challenges is a great start. Learn as much as you can, apply as much as you can, but don't stress the stress—or the things you did before you knew you were pregnant. Just commit to a conscious healthy pregnancy moving forward. As a friend of mine used to say, "If I could take back everything I did that was foolish, I wouldn't have any good stories to tell."

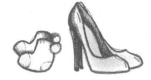

HOT MOM CHECKLIST: FOCUS ON THE THINGS YOU CAN CONTROL AND LET GO OF THE THINGS YOU CAN'T

Things you CAN control (with a little bit of help!):

❀ *Eat healthy.*

❀ *Take prenatal vitamins.*

❀ *Divide your body weight in half, and drink that many ounces of water per day.*

❀ *Limit caffeine.*

❀ *Reduce stress.*

❀ *Stop smoking.*

❀ *Stop drinking alcohol.*

Things you CAN"T control:

❀ *What you did prior to finding out you were pregnant*

❀ *Other people's reactions*

❀ *Other people's pregnancies*

❀ *How Angelina Jolie is having her next baby*

❀ *The grams of fat in chocolate truffles*

❀ *Your mother-in-law*

The "Perfect" Pregnancy

Perfect: (adj) Entirely without any flaws, defects, or short-comings.

You know those radiant maternity goddesses you see in the magazines? Or your preggie neighbor who is constantly going to morning yoga and afternoon Pilates? Or the mom-to-be who already has her child's name stitched in the uniforms for the day when he will take his spot at the ultimate preppy preschool? These moms may seem perfect, but they're not—they're just better at hiding their bad days. Everyone has rough patches and frustrations. That's the norm, especially during pregnancy. No one is perfect all the time, and no one relishes every day of her blessed nine-month event. Trust me. So relax. Accept that you can still be the person you have always been, with all your graces and foibles. Sometimes your breakfast will be rushed and not as healthy as you would like, and, try as you may, your boss/friend/mother-in-law will find a way to fray your last nerve.

I know it's hard, but—for your sanity—give up comparing yourself to others. You have no control over how your sister or your best friend is carrying her child. Give up focusing on why you're sick and she isn't, whether she's gained more or less weight than you, or if she has her baby's room finished already and you haven't even looked at a changing table. Focus on you and your pregnancy. Everyone finds her own joys and difficulties—so discover a way to balance for you, away from the perfection end of the spectrum.

Are You Talking to Me?

By twenty weeks, your unborn child hears and responds to sounds in his environment. The fetus can distinguish the rhythms and pitches of human voices clearly, and your voice is recognizable to your baby. So, although it may look a little silly, encourage your honey to talk to your belly every day—that way you'll both be sharing in the process and, when the baby is born, Dad can be a source of comfort too! My husband would talk to my belly and make up funny things he thought the baby would say in response. This always made me crack up.

It's never too early to start talking to your baby. In fact, it's said that a baby's heart rate drops when she or he hears the mother's voice soothing and comforting it.

A baby learns to associate sounds in the womb with sensations of comfort and discomfort. I know all the books tell you that listening to Mozart and other classical music will make your baby smarter . . . maybe.

"I'll never forget that moment after you were born; you were screaming and crying. The nurse bundled you up and handed you to your father. He started talking to you and immediately you stopped crying. Your eyes got wide, as if you were trying to focus on him. There was no doubt you knew his voice, and it had lulled you. That's all it took. In that second, your dad was hooked."
—My Mom

I'm equally in favor of Sarah McLachlan or Enya or U2. One thing I do know for sure is that you should be sure to listen to the music you like. When you hear sounds you enjoy, it sends a pleasing vibe to your mind, which circulates throughout your entire body. Your little passenger will be positively affected by your mood and the music. Also, nature sounds—like the ocean or running water—have a calming effect. Conversely, loud noises like yelling, barking dogs, and sirens can cause a baby to react. I went to see a James Bond movie in the theater when I was seven months pregnant. Oh man, it felt like I was viciously popping popcorn in my belly. We had to leave after only a few scenes.

You Are What You Eat . . .
Right Now Your Baby Is . . .
(Influenced, Anyway)

I've heard the umbilical cord called "a silent conversation between mother and child." It is the link through which you feed your baby and fill him or her with nutrients. Just as easily and quickly as you can deliver high-quality, nourishing foods, you can transport unhealthy food, air, water, etc., so it is more important than ever to watch and control what you ingest. While prenatal vitamins are your safety net, they are only a supplement. It is still crucial that you supply the vital nutrients found in a variety of foods such as fruits, vegetables, grains, eggs, nuts, fish, etc. to contribute toward your baby's healthy brain and body development. What's more, according to recent studies, our preferences for certain foods are a result of our genetics and how we were raised. By exposing your baby to various tastes in utero you help precondition him or her to eating them as a child and adult. You may be surprised to learn that babies have more taste buds before they are born than at any other time in their lives. Your little passenger is tasting and remembers all he or she comes in contact with. Preferences for vegetables or desserts are learned behaviors. So it has never been more important to get yourself on the right track with your diet; you are imprinting and influencing how your child is developing and how he or she will eat throughout life. The more informed you are about nutrition and healthy and yummy options, the better off you and your baby will be.

What the Heck Is "Organic" Anyway?

We have all heard the word *organic*. We know it signifies that a product is good for you, but why is it good for you? The answer is that labeling a food organic is essentially making a promise that the food you are eating is grown free of chemical fertilizers, pesticides, and insecticides, and it does not come from genetically modified seeds (GMOs). This is better for your body and better for the planet.

Organic meat means it comes from organically raised farm animals. They are treated in a more humane way, which protects their behavior and development, as well as the environment. Meat from grass-fed cattle tends to have five times the omega-3s and is leaner overall. Organic milk is produced free of antibiotics, pesticides, or artificial hormones. Organic and free-range hens are given space to lie down and walk around, unlike over 95 percent of the millions of chickens in the United States that are stacked in tight, tiny wire cages, squished on top of one another.

So toss the frozen TV dinners and processed foods (it is said the average American consumes about 150 pounds of processed food additives each year). Many processed meats like hot dogs are preserved with nitrates or nitrites (be sure to check the labels). Nitrates are water-soluble, so they can get into your bloodstream and pass to your baby. While the full effects of nitrates on the developing fetus are still unknown and being studied, nitrates and nitrites have been linked to various cancers and other ailments. Better be safe and stick to fresh chicken breast or organic turkey. If you are unsure about your diet, speak to your doctor and have him or her recommend a nutritionist who can work with you to create a delicious yet healthy menu.

Becoming a vegetarian is not recommended while you are pregnant. If you have been for years and are worried that you won't be able to continue your vegetarian or vegan diet, make sure you consult with your doctor. Let him or her know your dietary habits and concerns so that you can discuss adding protein and a variety of nutrients to your daily intake. Ask about additional supplements, and be sure to eat food rich in calcium and vitamin B12.

There are many cookbooks for vegetarians and vegans available. *The Vegetarian Mother's Cookbook: Whole foods to nourish pregnant and breastfeeding women—and their families* by Cathe Olson has over 300 recipes specifically designed for the pregnant and lactating mother.

BUMP ON A BUDGET

Plant a garden and grow your own organic food. If you don't have a yard, use your windowsill to grow fresh herbs.

ECO-MINDED MAMA

Buy fruits and vegetables in season. They are more likely to be grown locally and will contain fewer chemicals; as produce reaches the end of its peak season, farmers have to use more chemicals to keep it from rotting. Rinse all produce in water before eating, especially if it is not labeled organic. This will remove some of the pesticide residue on its surface.

Something's Fishy. . . .

Eating the right type of fish during pregnancy is a great and healthy way to get your share of important omega-3s. However, some fish have high levels of mercury and can damage your baby's immune system and brain development. To be safe, stay away from raw fish and sushi, canned tuna, oysters, sea bass, halibut, and grouper.

Salmon is excellent, either wild or canned. Sardines, anchovies, trout, shrimp, scallops, mahimahi, catfish, crab, flounder, haddock are all great seafood choices that are low in contaminants. Make sure to buy fresh, and when in doubt, talk to your doctor. I know I always say that, but these are just guidelines; your doctor knows your body and your individual pregnancy, so he or she will be able to tailor a diet for you based on your specific needs.

So Cheesy

Eating unpasteurized or soft cheeses is not a good idea during pregnancy, as they can harbor a bacteria called *Listeria*. While it has little to no effect on adults, it can be dangerous to fetuses, so avoid Brie, goat cheese, feta, etc., until after the baby is born. Don't worry: hard cheese like American or Swiss, as well as cream cheese, cottage cheese, and yogurt, are fine.

If eating healthy is not already part of your routine, there are simple ways to start integrating healthier foods. There has never been a better time to get yourself on the right track, and you will feel good knowing you are giving your baby the best start possible. Besides, you will have more energy yourself. The easiest way to upgrade your diet is to start substituting whole wheat bread for white, eating whole grain cereals instead of anything sugary (whole grains are said to help settle a queasy stomach). Add leafy greens, vegetables, and fruits (fresh or dried) wherever and whenever possible. Beans are a great source of protein and will boost your energy. I add black beans to my scrambled eggs in the morning. Pinto beans or red beans taste delicious on a salad, cannellini beans can add flavor to any pasta. Be sure to eat small meals throughout the day to keep your blood sugar regulated and energy up. When I was pregnant I always had water, energy bars, and trail mix in my purse.

Does This Fetus
Make Me Look Fat?

The fact that *pregorexia* (preoccupation with staying thin during maternity and feeling uncomfortable with the normal and natural weight gain that comes with a healthy pregnancy) is even a word is frightening. If you think that it only affects women who have battled with anorexia or bulemia, you are mistaken, though women with eating disorders are more at risk. A wave of thin celebrity moms with perfect couture baby bumps are said to have fueled this new mind-set of women who brag that they can still fit into their jeans in the second trimester or that they "hardly look pregnant." Now, it is challenging for any woman to pack on extra pounds and experience changes in the shape and look of her body—I get it—but when you are pregnant, you should look pregnant. It's beautiful and normal, and there is nothing glamorous about malnutrition or putting your baby at risk for birth defects. A pregorexic puts at risk not only her baby's health but her own as well; remember, the body will protect its growing baby at the expense of the mother. If you eat healthy and exercise moderately, you will fill out just right and bounce back easier. Your preoccupation in pregnancy should be with the baby you are carrying, not your waistline. So if you struggled with eating disorders in your youth, or recognize yourself in this paragraph, you should inform your doctor right away so that he can pay extra attention to your diet and recommend people to talk to and counsel you so you are getting adequate emotional support.

Seeing the Big Picture

Even the things we see can have a positive or negative effect on our little passengers. Remember human beings are very visual creatures, and our interpretations of what we see can influence our sense of comfort or discomfort. When you look at children playing or lovers kissing, it evokes a positive feeling inside you. In contrast, when you see violent imagery, it produces negative emotions. In other words, opt for the romantic comedy over the horror flick.

So what are the Hot Mom "key words" for creating a positive physical and mental connection to your baby? Keep calm, take care of your body and mind, have a little fun, and—most of all—keep a positive mind-set.

ECO-MINDED MAMA

Plant a tree when you find out you're pregnant. You can watch it grow as your belly grows. It will make you feel good, and once your baby is older, you can take care of it together.

Sonogram = Ultrasound = Ultracool

Speaking of amazing sights, seeing the ultrasound for the first time ranks up there as a truly magical experience. When the doctor projects that image onto the screen, it can resemble something out of a spin art machine.

At our first ultrasound, we stared at the fuzzy black-and-white photo of a fuzzy lima bean in awe. My husband, Bryan, looked at me and said jokingly, "I think it looks like me." Truthfully, whether your baby resembles a cashew or a raisin, she or he is yours, and the moment you first see the baby is full of sheer pride that only parents can feel.

"They rub what looks like a pricing gun over your wife's belly until you get a picture so grainy you are too embarrassed to admit that, to you, what you are looking at could either be a baby or a police artist's depiction of the Pillsbury Dough-boy accidentally heated in a microwave."
—Michael Crider, from The Guy's Guide to Surviving Pregnancy, Childbirth, and the First Year of Fatherhood

Gabe's dad was over the moon from the start. I could have sworn I heard him ask the doctor for wallet-sized photos of the ultrasound. He couldn't wait to show off his blob.

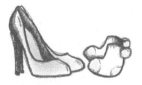

Images by Ellyn (www.imagesbyellyn.net) has beautiful frames specially designed with sweet and funny sayings and sized to show off your ultrasound photo.

MY FAVORITES INCLUDE

✿ "A miracle waiting to be seen . . ."

✿ "First time I ever saw your face . . ."

✿ "Love at First Sight"

✿ "Under Construction"

✿ "It's a Jungle in Here"

Create a nickname for your little embryo and use it all the time; it will help bond you. After my first ultrasound, we referred to ours as the "Little Lima Bean" because that was our first impression of the adorable little spot on the screen. Other names I've heard include Smudge, Moose, Tripod, Blinky, and Dynamo.

Once we learned we were expecting not one but two babies, we knew we would have significant fun with in-utero nicknames. However, we held off on using them until we knew what variety of genitals we were dealing with in there. After we got the full-frontal view of each via ultrasound, the pairings were never ending. Fred and Wilma. Lucy and Ricky. Bonnie and Clyde. Bill and Hillary. Of course, many of those monikers were bandied about based on their activity level and intensity at any given moment. From whence my beloved husband extracted these names, I may never know, but when we actually spoke of or referred to them as our own offspring (and not infamous couples from our pop-cultural lexicon), they were Cornbread and Loomis. Used in a sentence? Come on, Cornbread and Loomis, we're off to the Prepared Childbirth class.

—Cheryl Lage,
mommy to Darren and Sarah
and author of *Twinspiration*

JOURNAL—MONTH TWO

(Don't skip this part, you'll thank me later!)

1. What healthy foods did you eat today?

_____

_____

_____

_____

_____

_____

_____

_____

_____

_____

_____

_____

_____

_____

_____

_____

_____

_____

2. List the songs that you use to bring you back to earth.

_____

_____

_____

_____

_____

_____

_____

_____

_____

_____

_____

_____

_____

_____

_____

_____

_____

_____

_____

3. What's your baby's womb nickname?

_____

_____

_____

_____

_____

_____

_____

_____

4. Write down a talk you've had with your baby. Make up her or his side of the conversation!

_____

_____

_____

_____

_____

_____

_____

_____

_____

_____

5. What are your favorite feel-good movies? Make a plan to see them over the next eight months.

_____

_____

_____

_____

_____

_____

_____

_____

_____

_____

_____

_____

_____

_____

_____

_____

_____

_____

_____

_____

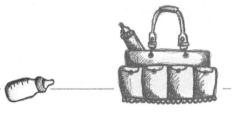

Three

"You Don't Have Childbearing Hips"

The moment the second line on the pee stick turns pink,
women discover they've entered a world of parenting experts.
Friends, family, colleagues, the UPS delivery guy . . .
suddenly everybody is a trove of advice.

—Stefanie Wilder-Taylor,
author of *Sippy Cups Are Not for Chardonnay*

The Weird, the Horrific, and the Occasionally Helpful: Pregnancy Tales

"You don't have childbearing hips." "If you crave Doritos, you're going to have a boy." Why is it that as soon as people find out you're pregnant, they feel obligated to share all their often useless, odd, and sometimes downright scary stories and advice? Sure, it comes from a good place, but it's a little disconcerting when you're in line at the movies and the woman behind you shares how, in her ninth month, she managed to shave her legs without being able to see them. (That was actually very practical advice, which I did follow.) But once in a while, I got caught up by a storyteller's absolute conviction and got carried away, no matter how tall the tale. It was my first child; what did I know? Someone who birthed and raised three children should know about these things, right?

To help you sort out the fact from the fiction, let me offer the following guide:

❁ If you are carrying in front and low, you are having a boy. Hey, I carried in front and low, and I had a boy. Hmm.

❁ If you crave salty food, you are having a boy, and if you crave sweets, you're having a girl. Now, I craved everything: sweet, salty, organic, processed . . . not sure how that fits.

❁ If your skin is breaking out, you know it is most likely going to be a girl; well, I broke out worse than a teenager . . . so I wouldn't bank on this one.

❁ If your husband puts on weight during your pregnancy, you are having a girl! My husband didn't gain a pound, and we had a boy.

❁ If you have heartburn, your baby will be born with a lot of hair. HA! I had terrible

heartburn, and my son was as bald as an
eagle for his first year and a half.

✿ And if you're seeing little green men? Well,
that has nothing to do with pregnancy, but
you should see your shrink.

The Mayans ("old wives" from hundreds of years
ago) determined the sex of a baby by calculating the
mother's age at conception (that's twenty-four for me)
and the year of the birth (1999). If both are even or
odd, then the baby is a girl. If one is even and the other
odd, then the baby will be a boy. Now, this calculation
was absolutely correct for me—but it might not be a
predictor for you. The only thing you know for sure is
that you will have a BABY, and almost everyone you
meet will have a comment or idea about your child's
potential gender, eye color, disposition, and future ability on the soccer field.

Why do these myths survive? Why did I, a rational,
twenty-first-century woman, believe some of them?
Simple. It's fifty-fifty odds! When's the last time you had
that in Vegas! The women who have boys after accidentally eating a spider boast for the rest of their lives, "Yes,
it's true, spiders produce boys." And the ones who don't
have a boy? Well, they forget about the whole thing, stay
quiet, and chalk it up as an old wives' tale. It's a case of
she who speaks loudest creates the most myths.

Let the games begin. Baby pools are a fun way to
heighten the anticipation and incorporate those around
you into the experience. Friends, relatives, and colleagues can guess on the date, size, sex, and weight of
the baby. The pot can go to the winner, to the parents,

to the baby, or split between all three. Check out www.
pregpool.com.

Oh, the Horror . . .

There should be some sort of a study done to find out
what compels women to tell you their "labor and pregnancy horror stories." I firmly believe there should be
a law that prohibits scaring the "you-know-what" out
of expecting moms. Mournful tales of hours in labor,
medical mysteries, bodily fluids in odd places . . . well,
when you're already on the trip, you can't get off the
train, so you're stuck carrying these images with you.
Maybe you can consider these stories as worst-case scenarios and fully believe that what you experience will
be at least 90 percent better! Also, remember many of
these stories may be a bit, um . . . exaggerated. Let's
face it; it sounds a bit more impressive to say that you
endured an unbearable thirty-eight hours of labor than,
say, four hours with drugs and a back massager.

Better brace yourself; horror stories will come at
you when you least expect it. You may find yourself,
like I did, innocently buying groceries when a cashier
will notice your belly and proceed to tell you in graphic
detail about her twenty-nine hours of labor, how she
pushed and pushed and experienced the most excruciating pain in her life. I just wanted to buy a few bananas
and some ketchup but instead came home with a bag
full of panic. The images she conjured up stayed with

me for days. If I could have run away, I would have, but I was held hostage—the woman had my snacks! So if someone starts to tell you her or his story and it sounds like it's going to take a bad turn, do your best to change the subject or immediately excuse yourself to go to the bathroom. You're pregnant; you always have to pee. And once you're by yourself, repeat this mantra: "I am going to deliver with ease; my birth will be quick and painless." Positive thinking works.

The Pregnancy Police

Almost as bad as the people who tell you all the gory details of their delivery are the people who want to "inform" you of all the things you are doing wrong, should be doing, or should stay away from. Beware, the Pregnancy Police are out in full force, where you least expect them, and they are always ready to offer you (inflict upon you) a tip or tale to "help." This is a little trickier, because their "advice" actually sounds relevant to things in our world today—not myths from the Old Country, but stories right out of your environment. You know, "That wickedly spicy salad dressing from X Restaurant will instigate labor," or, "Stay away from power lines," and better yet, "Synthetic fabrics cause allergies in newborns." Most of these myths concern the possible effects of certain foods we're likely to eat, or technology we're bound to encounter, or the physical activities that we always look forward to. But if you cut out everything these stories and people warn you about, you'd spend your pregnancy sitting in a wooden chair, eating boiled applesauce, talking to friends on a rotary phone.

Remember, moderation and a bit of rational thought can guide you through most pregnancy dilemmas, and, if you have any questions about some questionable advice, there are many expert sources available in person, on the web, or in your library. But just so you're acquainted with the territory, here are four pregnancy myths that continue to prevail. You be the judge!

1. *You shouldn't exercise while pregnant.* While triathlons and marathons aren't a good idea during pregnancy, moderate exercise is good for your physical and mental health. As always, consult your doctor when beginning an exercise routine, and let your body be your guide. Moving with the lump actually can feel good!

2. *Using a computer, microwave, or cell phone may stress the baby or cause premature birth.* You will hear these warnings for sure! Some people are adamant that invisible energy waves affect pregnancy. Others say tests prove otherwise. There is a lot of conflicting evidence out there. This is territory where your own beliefs will come strongly into play.

3. *You shouldn't travel at all during pregnancy.* In general, up until about thirty-four weeks, you should feel free to travel just as if you're

not pregnant. After that, you risk going into labor.

4. *Having sex will hurt our baby.* Hello, ladies! Don't deprive yourself of some physical joy and loving consideration. If you have a low-risk pregnancy, there is no need for skipping sex unless it's personally uncomfortable. Then you might consider your favorite physical intimacy alternatives. You might be advised to avoid sex if you have had a history of preterm labor or are going through a high-risk pregnancy. Let your doctor be the judge if you have any concerns.

Take all the stories and warnings in stride and take a deep breath, look past the insanity, and find the humor. So when the woman in Target tells you that it looks like your left boob is bigger than your right and that means you'll be having a boy (this happened to a friend of mine), you can laugh.

Seriously, with the Internet and so many ways to access information, moms-to-be are more educated today than ever. Unlike me, you are probably too hip to fall for any of those old pregnancy myths. But first-time moms can still be susceptible and vulnerable, so if someone tells you not to take a bath because you might drown the baby or expose your child to water-germs, activate your intuition and check a few sources. Finally, if someone cautions you about delivery success based on the size of your "non-childbearing" hips, tell them to take a hike!

Childbearing Hips!?!

Now, I don't have "childbearing hips," as they say. I have, as my mom called them, snake hips or no hips. I have always been petite with a small frame. Even at twenty-four, my body resembled a thirteen-year-old girl's more than that of a woman months away from giving birth. My frame didn't look like it could support a backpack, let alone an eight-pound baby. From the time I found out I was pregnant, my mother-in-law was deeply—and I mean deeply—concerned because I didn't have "childbearing hips." "You are just so tiny, I don't know how you'll get a baby out" . . . and so on, and, oh so often. I actually started to worry: What if my pelvis wasn't designed for giving birth? What if I was in for extreme back and birth pain? What if I was destined for an emergency C-section?

Attitudes are infectious. Luckily my doctor assured me that the size of my hips had no bearing on the difficulty of my delivery. He told me that I would be just fine, that I would have a smooth and easy delivery. I loved my doctor. He had a way of making me feel so at ease, so calm. Never once did I doubt that I would have a smooth delivery, because Dr. Z told me I would. He was the best, with a wall of plaques, awards, and fancy titles to prove it. The positive vibe was reinforced by the nurses in his office. "Yes, all of his patients have easy deliveries." Was it some sort of magic? Maybe. I now realize that it had more to do with his ability to calm his patients and get them to focus on the positive and on their own strengths. Our confidence in him gave us the confidence to believe in ourselves.

Our minds are awfully powerful, and our minds and bodies are connected. The more we energize something with our thoughts, the more we increase the chances of its happening, good or bad. Dwelling on your fear of not having big enough hips to push out your baby or having to have a Cesarean or experiencing unbearable pain will only prolong the torture and, ironically, may cause it to come about!

When I announced I was pregnant for the first time, my mother-in-law said, "Whatever you do, don't have the baby during the Super Bowl. We have had a party for the last twenty years, and there will be lots of out-of-town guests." I sort of laughed and dismissed her comment. But sure enough, my water broke during the kickoff of the Super Bowl game! When someone puts something in your mind, your body just can't help but make the offhanded comment come true! Just for the record, both of my children were born the morning after Super Bowl Sunday. How is that for the power of thought?
　　—Hilary J. Probst, mom of two, teacher, and Hot Moms Club member

A Few Myths
That Have a Grain of Truth

There are a few old stories that have a real bearing on pregnancy, and most of these have to do with eating foods that have a chance of being contaminated. I'm sure your doctor has given you the list of foods and activities to avoid, but it bears repeating:

- ❀ Forget shellfish and raw meat or eggs.

- ❀ Put down the Jägermeister—and any other alcoholic beverages.

- ❀ Say good-bye to exotic unpasteurized soft cheese. (Ah, au revoir, Brie . . . at least for now!)

- ❀ Skip the sauna.

- ❀ Get someone else to empty the cat box.

- ❀ Don't rent *Rosemary's Baby* or *Alien II*!

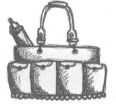

A Few Words of Advice on Advice-Givers

Women always love to share their point of view of what time of day is best to take prenatal vitamins, why doulas are a must-have or not, whether to bare your belly, and why one cup of coffee is absolutely deadly (or in my case lifesaving!). . . . The list goes on and on. There are so many decisions to make about pregnancy and motherhood, and every woman obviously convinces herself which way is best for her.

Of course, as women we want to help others, so that's why so many women offer so many "fabulous" suggestions, which are often really just reinforcements of their own past decisions. So when you receive unsolicited advice, I've found the best response is to understand that the women offering it may have some sort of subconscious (albeit well-intentioned) agenda. Thank them politely, mention you'll give it a try, and move on. Everyone's happy.

—Kristen Moss,
mom of two and Hot Moms Club member

I think advice is great, and I suggest becoming as informed as possible, but please don't buy into everything you're told. From the moment we conceive, we become instinctually maternal. Everyone has a different pregnancy experience, but YOU alone are the best judge of what is ultimately the best thing for you and your baby. Not your mother or your cousin Rita who has had six kids in six years—You. Trust that.

Now, for those of you who have developed a two-pack-a-day saltine habit due to intense nausea and "morning" sickness, you are the exception to the advice rule. Please take any guidance, suggestions, opinions, or "always works!" remedies from ANYONE who might help you feel better.

FACT

66 to 80 percent of women experience some nausea in the first trimester.

80 percent of them have nausea that lasts all day.

Queen Yak

I was lucky; I didn't get sick during my pregnancy. Some friends who did say nothing helped (sorry). What works for one mom may not work for another. Here is a list of things the majority of moms said worked best. Test out a few and see what combination works for you—and if you have a trick or secret remedy, please log onto our website (www.hotmomsclub.com) and share it!

- ❀ Take more vitamin B6 (scientifically proven to help with nausea and keep hormonal balance).

- ❀ Try B-natal TheraPops—cherry-flavored lollipops loaded with B6 and sugar.

- ❀ Morning Sickness Magic is an herbal remedy with ginger, B6, red raspberry leaf, and folic acid. It has no artificial flavors or colors and is FDA approved.

- ❀ Munch on some ginger or suck ginger-flavored candies.

- ❀ Squeeze a little lemon juice on your wrists.

- ❀ Stay cool. Heat increases nausea.

- ❀ Eat plain salted crackers first thing in the morning (many moms keep them by the bed).

- ❀ Get more sleep. You are more likely to feel sick when you are tired.

- ❀ Do not drink fluids with your meals.

❁ Avoid spicy meals and fried foods or anything with a strong odor.

❁ Take prenatal vitamins later in the day or
before bed.

The only thing more horrifying than hurling into your toilet is finding yourself in public asking a complete stranger for a tissue as you wipe spitup from your mouth. Morning Chicness Bags (www.morningchicnessbags.com) are basically those airplane barf bags but with pretty feminine designs. It's smart to keep a few in your purse, along with mints, hand sanitizer, and some wipes, so just in case your wave of nausea gets *ugly* . . .

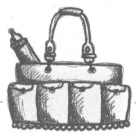

Olympic Freestyle Vomiting

The Technicolor yawn, yakking, hurling, spewing chunks, blowing chow, ralphing, praying to the porcelain goddess. So many cute collegiate euphemisms dedicated to a digestive encore. Anthropologists say that in order to judge the value a particular society places on a subject, simply count the number of words used to describe it. I'm going to defend my singular obsession with vomiting. My very survival depends on trying to find meaning and variety in the purgatory of morning, noon, night, and whatever's-in-between sickness. I'm coming to the end of my first trimester, and there's no relief in sight. Generally I vomit about once a day, not too bad. But I devote the rest of the day trying to avoid a repeat performance. I desperately want what little food I choke down to stay down. Don't talk to me about saltines, pretzels, protein in any form, mint tea, lemon sniffing, potato chips, or any other lame-ass remedies. I've tried them all, and they don't work for me.

The only thing that does work is eating something constantly. But whatever that something is, it has to be orange colored. Cheetos, baby carrots, grilled cheese sandwiches, orange slices, McDonald's Hi-C Orange drink sipped through that fat striped orange straw, and pumpkin pie. The color orange is truly magical, and I didn't read that in any stupid book. However, there's a strong likelihood that my baby will be born with the skin tone of an Oompa-Loompa.

To maintain a questionable level of sanity, I have devised an Olympic-style scoring system to rate my vomiting performance. I know, I know, too much time on my hands. And you know what? You're right. Ever since morning sickness set in, I've become debilitated. I have spent days just being horizontal and watching bad TV. I watched lots of the Olympics when they were on, and the seeds of madness implanted themselves into my glucose-deprived brain. Watching gymnastics and platform diving, I began to see a parallel between athletics and vomiting. Both are intensely physical performances with a strong mental component. Both demand rigorous commitment to the moment. And both can be scored with similar criteria of speed, form, and accuracy. Here is my scoring system for Olympic Freestyle Vomiting:

1. Speed. How fast do I make it to the toilet when the need arises? Now here, the DISMOUNT from the bed, couch, or whatever is crucial. A clean dismount can make the difference between a mess to clean up or a simple flush of the toilet. That means no legs entangled in blankets, no tripping, no flailing about. A clean dismount consists of both feet landing securely on the floor and a quick sprint to the nearest commode.

2. Form. This is also crucial to a high-scoring vomiting routine. Proper form exhibits flexibility and grace. Point deductions for kneeling or using your hands to brace yourself against the toilet. Optimum form consists of a standing posture with knees slightly bent and head as close to toilet bowl as possible to minimize unsightly splash back. Extra points awarded if toilet seat is up and one hand holds hair back from face. Other judges may differ on this, but if you're going to all the trouble, why not make it pretty?

3. Accuracy. Only a bull's-eye into the dead center of the toilet can bring home the gold. Scores decrease as proximity from toilet bowl increases. Although accuracy is undoubtedly its own acquired skill, without proper speed and form, it is nearly impossible.

These are my guidelines for what it takes to be a champion vomiter, after much painstaking training and practice. I like to think that I've elevated my pregnancy to another level of human endurance. I don't think it will ever catch on as a spectator sport, but with synchronized swimming and trampoline being recognized, I suppose anything's possible. I hope to be in retirement, but something tells me I'll be the reluctant torchbearer for a while longer.

—Minsun Park,
SheKnows columnist and mom of two

I'll Have Some Pickles, Ice Cream, and Anchovies on That, Please

You may be experiencing some strong cravings: mango and peanut butter and artichoke sandwiches or entire slabs of chocolate cake or Cheetos on ice cream. During my pregnancy, I had to have soft scrambled eggs with cheese, spinach, tomato, and onion every day. And, did I mention, with pure maple syrup glopped on top? I am not kidding; it was a ritual. Oh, and I couldn't look at a salad without getting disgusted and annoyed. I didn't meet a salad that didn't literally offend me. Who knows what my body needed from that particular combination, but it seemed to help me and my baby. Most often doctors say to follow your cravings and trust your body. Unless of course, you, like some pregnant women, are craving paint chips or laundry starch (it's true!). In that case, check with your physician.

Cravings are fine as long as the rest of your diet is still in order. We've all made resolutions to "eat better," and there's still plenty of opportunity to move toward that optimum healthy diet while you're pregnant. What better time is there than now? Remember, the nutrients that you provide are helping your little one grow. Enlist the spouse to get your favorite fruits and vegetables, discover a new way to grill or broil your favorite protein source (only you know whether that's vegan or carnivore or somewhere in-between), and find ways to indulge that are healthy.

Häagen-Dazs Five ice cream line contains only five natural ingredients. Flavors include mint, ginger, coffee, vanilla bean, passion fruit, brown sugar, and milk chocolate. Something for every craving without the guilt!!!

My weird cravings ended up being "cruel and unusual punishment" for my husband! My random and sometimes shocking snacks ranged from Froot Loops with a side of Coco Puffs to just plain ol' bacon—deep fried! Or how about a midnight nibble on extra-garlicky Italian breadsticks in bed? My poor best friend was the slave to my appetite. Overnight he went from my husband to the "official food fetcher." It wasn't an easy job, as my cravings were in full swing around the clock. In addition, I couldn't get all the food in my mouth fast enough! His duty to find the food to satiate my hunger was not an easy one. It wasn't as simple as "Honey, I would like some ice cream." I had multidimensional desires from my stomach and mouth. It was more like "Honey, I would like some bubble gum ice cream with homemade whipped cream and some sprinkles on top!"

—Jennifer Nicole Lee,
fitness expert and life coach

"I Gotta Pee" Card

When cornered by unsolicited advice or delivery war stories or just that crazy neighbor down the street, don't hesitate to excuse yourself to the nearest restroom. Remember, pregnant women always have to go; this is your foolproof way out of any conversation. You could also fake like you're getting sick. Both are equally effective!

Blame It on the Dog

Since your first symptoms of pregnancy, if you're like me, you may have had some, uh, interesting special effects. Bloating, burping, and farting are by-products of progesterone, so there's no getting around an increase in gas manufacturing during pregnancy. In addition, you have a person growing inside of you who takes up room, which puts pressure on your digestive system, and presto!—you're the life of the party.

Passing gas like a truck driver will no doubt make you a hero with the seven-year-old boys. Or, if you have young children, you will be somewhat of a star for burping and farting louder than the characters on *South Park*—but other than the grammar school set, you are out of luck. What to do? You can carry a small dog in your purse, or you can follow some simple steps to reduce the pressure:

1. Drink more water.

2. Avoid gassy foods like cabbage, beans, and onions.

3. Eat smaller meals—and eat slower!

4. Keep an eye out for the nearest ladies' room!

"I'm Not an Idiot, I'm Pregnant!"

Another wonderful side effect of pregnancy that you can spin to your advantage is that it actually makes you dumb. Yup, you heard correct; it's called Pregnancy Brain, also known as Baby Brain Drain or Placenta Brain. That's right, they have an official name for the reason why you can't ever seem to find your keys or remember your own name or how you went a whole day wearing two different shoes without noticing. It's simple forgetfulness, short-term memory loss, and temporary confusion all rolled into one. Some doctors say it's a myth, but the moms I've talked to all agree it is very real. Now, since forgetfulness is a permanent condition of mine, it was hard to tell if this affected me or not, but I will say this—had I known about it and all of the fancy official names, I would have certainly called it to my defense. So next time instead of saying, "Oh, silly me, I'm such a ding dong. I pulled into the neighbor's driveway again," try saying, "You'll have to excuse me, my brain is on temporary loan to my baby."

I have the worst pregnancy brain! I found my phone in the pantry, my husband finds phones I left in the fridge. I went with my husband to go on a date, we laughed as I learned I put the (home) phone in my pocket on the way out. I try to make little notes for myself, and that helps . . . but not really. I've been very forgetful lately. And it's not fair the second time around! I can't play the pregnancy card with my husband. He just doesn't buy it!
—actress Soleil Moon Frye,
Hot Moms Club partner and
owner of The Little Seed baby store

Sometimes Being a Hot Mom Is Knowing When to Stay Cool

To review: no pregnancy escapes old wives' tales. It's part of the experience, I guess. Our bodies are changing in so many ways that it's confusing, and turning to others for help is natural. And it's natural for others to want to offer their experience and love, even if it is misinformed or completely dysfunctional. It may be helpful to remember that words are just that—words. You can make the decision on how they will affect you and if they will affect you. Find ways to stay cool when you feel your inside worry rising! With that in mind, whenever you hear dubious wisdom:

1. *Listen, but don't react.* Focus on the person and her intent, not on the advice.

2. *Do your own research* (can you say Google?). If something sounds probable, check out three other sources. Aren't you feeling more comfortable already?

3. *Ask the other man or woman . . . your doctor.* Most often, she or he has heard it all before and can guide you to the truth.

4. *Keep your sense of humor.* A pregnant friend of mine would counter people's stories with even more outrageous ones, like "brushing your teeth when pregnant causes hairy babies" and "cravings for sweets means your child will like unicorns." And then she'd swear they were true without even cracking a smile!

Create Your Own Pregnancy Story

What a great idea! Turn all your positive Hot Mom energy to creating a positive, relaxed story for your child-to-be's journey. Words and images can work in positive ways, and as a Hot Mom, you can visualize your pregnancy as one where you are still your fabulous self, just a bit slowed down and a bit more aware. You're not a princess locked in a castle but a modern woman with your own strengths and quirks on an exciting (and, for you, uncharted) voyage.

And it's never too early to start your visualizations of labor. I continually saw myself delivering with ease. I would repeat to myself, "I am going to push this baby out without a problem." No matter what anyone told me about the impending pain, I continually told myself, "I can handle anything that comes my way" and "I will have the strength and courage of a warrior." Say whatever works for you. Just keep it focused on the positive.

Use mantras to combat any fears you have during your pregnancy or any people who try to worry or stress you out. As it turned out, I had no problems. I delivered a healthy baby boy—quickly and with ease! Mantras, affirmations, and visualizations are powerful. I use them in all areas of my life . . . and they work. My favorite mantra for pregnancy? "I will have a quick and easy delivery of a beautiful, healthy baby!"

Doin' the Mood Swing

It's not only other people who may get under your skin during pregnancy. Remember how you would blame PMS for all of your emotional or angry moments? Well, now you can blame pregnancy hormones—the supersized version of PMS. Sure, it's natural to start sobbing in the middle of Pottery Barn because the new colors are just so beautiful and literally the next minute feeling like you want to drop kick the sales guy for saying hello. Sure. As you may know by now, these crazy mood swings are common during pregnancy. They are especially strong in the first trimester, but they continue throughout. These ups and downs are all a natural part of the hormonal tidal flows surging through your body—those bursts of chemicals that are helping your baby grow but that are not the norm for your metabolism (or your spouse's). These surges are also amplified by uncomfortable sensations in your body, worries about your pregnancy, and the emotional revolution in your lifestyle. Talk about learning to surf on the big waves.

There are several different suggestions for maintaining a more even keel: pregnancy vitamins, particularly B6; reducing sugar intake; and regular sleep. All of these are extremely helpful. But there is one thing I know for sure. trying to stop a mood swing in progress is like trying to stop an erupting volcano. Still, you can always try: in the moment, it's hard to believe that your emotions aren't real or rational, but if you can activate a small bit of awareness and a sense of humor right when you feel an overwhelming urge to gush, cry, scream, or laugh (beyond your norm), sometimes you can stop the Vesuvius Condition! Learning to soothe yourself now when you feel anxious, stressed, or emotional will certainly help you as you are raising your kids, and many of these techniques work well in relaxing your little ones as well.

SOME TIPS ON TAMING YOUR MOM-TO-BE MOOD SWINGS

❀ Make music your best friend. Create a CD or a play list of songs guaranteed to make you smile or calm you down any time you start feeling emotional.

❁ Breathe deeply. Listen to yourself inhale and exhale. (I use this with my son when he is on the verge of a meltdown. Having him focus on breathing in and out really distracts him.)

❁ Taking a minute to count to ten and back down again before you react tends to take a little of the edge off. (This tip not only works for me today but I have also taught my son to count to ten and back again when he is about to get worked up about something, and it's amazing what a difference in reaction that little bit of time and shift of focus can make.)

Hormones did a number on my emotions when I was pregnant, and one night I literally threw myself on my bed weeping into my pillow because TiVo had not taped *The Amazing Race*. I could not control the sobs for upward of twenty minutes. And the tears flowed for most of the night. My husband, Dave, was really good about it, though surprised at first. He managed to keep his laughter hidden from me, and by bedtime, I was laughing (still crying) at myself. I had cried so hard that the next morning I woke up with burst blood vessels! I still get teased about it!

—Alison Sweeney,
mom of two, *Days of Our Lives* actress,
and host of *The Biggest Loser*

BYOB (Bring Your Own Boob or Bottle)

About now, another barrage of advice is coming about birthing and breastfeeding. I am not really sure why women get so heated over this, but it seems that this is a passionate debate. There is no doubt about the advantages to breastfeeding your baby. In a boxing match between the nutrients of the mother (which are tailor-made for your specific child) and generic formula (which is, well, generic), breast milk wins hands down. However, breastfeeding is not for everyone. You may not want to—or you may not be able to. And that's okay. For what it's worth, my mom didn't breastfeed me or my brother and sister, and we turned out just fine. My sister never saw a B in her life—she graduated from Penn State with high honors and has received several master's degrees. So if you fear Junior's shot at Harvard is over because you can't lactate . . . sleep easier tonight.

Breastfeeding is a lot harder than it looks. I swear I aced the classes, but Gabe and I just couldn't get it down. I wanted him to have the breast milk. So-o-o—I pumped. It was a joke. For a petite person, I had pumped enough milk to feed a small country. I would pump so much that I had to freeze the extra. My mom posted a sign saying Jessie's Milking Parlor over the rocker and machine. My son was drinking breast milk for weeks after I stopped pumping. I have to admit that at first I was disappointed that we couldn't breastfeed, but I really liked feeding him a bottle. I also liked watching my husband, my dad, my mom, my brother, etc., feed him—and I know they loved it too. That's not to mention how much I appreciated it when my parents were visiting and they took turns getting up at night with the baby; that was so nice. The bottom line: it's your decision. Get all the facts. And it's okay if you change your mind afterward. You have to do what's best for you. No pressure.

BUMP ON A BUDGET

Formula for one baby can cost $1,500 to $8,000 dollars a year. If you can do it, breastfeeding is clearly the economical way to go!

ECO-MINDED MAMA

Circumstances sometimes make breastfeeding impossible, and although there isn't a formula that can compare to or be substituted for breast milk, there are formula brands that offer organic choices and have DHA, a key nutrient found in breast milk. Parent's Choice (www.parentschoiceformula.com) and Bright Beginnings (www.brightbeginnings.com) both have organic formula with DHA. Similac (www.similacorganic.com) is the first major formula company to offer an organic version of its formula.

Adiri Natural Nurser baby bottles (www.adiri.com) provide a sensory experience that comes close to breastfeeding. They are perfect for weaning little ones off the bottle or creating an intimate and natural first feeding experience for those moms who can't or don't wish to breastfeed. BornFree bottles (www.newbornfree.com) have a system that helps with colic. They are eco-friendly and BPA-free (no chemicals).

Booby Trap

Shari Criso is a certified nurse midwife, board-certified lactation consultant, and proud mother of two daughters, whom she success-fully breastfed. Through her learning center, the Birth Boutique (www.birthboutique.com), Shari helps educate, empower, and inspire thousands of new moms to successfully breast-feed. This is her advice for Hot Moms-to-be.

Breastfeeding is simple, but usually not easy! Wanting a happy, healthy, thriving baby is an instinct; knowing how to achieve that is a learned skill. Most moms think breastfeed-ing is natural and are usually shocked when it doesn't just come easily. They expect to just put the baby to the breast and the baby will just know what to do. For most people, this couldn't be further from the truth. The hardest time for mom is usually the first four weeks (getting through the hospital, recover-ing from the birth, engorgement, etc.). It's all about getting over that "hump"! As with any new skill, it takes practice, and luckily, that is what you will be doing—practicing a lot!!

Just like breastfeeding, pregnancy and birth are also natural, but you would never go through your pregnancy without prenatal care and childbirthing classes. You would never deliver at home unattended and just assume you had some genetic condition when you had a bad outcome!! Why would you expect breastfeeding to be any different?

That's why it is superimportant for all expectant parents to prepare for breastfeeding by purchasing the essential equipment they will need and attending or watching a breastfeeding class prior to the arrival of their baby. Most expectant mothers do not take a class and expect the nurses to teach them once they get to the hospital. This usually does not work out well, since the nurses have many patients to attend to and may have limited or contradictory knowledge of breastfeeding. What's more, you are usually discharged before your milk even comes in!

It is also critical for dads to be involved in the learning process. Studies show that one of the most important factors for success with breastfeeding is a supportive partner. Too many breastfeeding classes do not include dad, which I think is a big mistake! Fathers can offer the necessary support and even help with breastfeeding when you are the only ones home alone together after your baby is born. Breastfeeding is a team effort. You may be the one with the breasts, but feeding and nurturing your new baby requires partnership!

Not only is our species capable of breastfeeding; as mammals we are actually defined by it (**def:** any of a class of warm-blooded higher vertebrates that nourish their young with milk). Learning the necessary skills is the first step, building your confidence and really committing to this amazing gift for your baby is what will ensure your success!

MOTHER KNOWS BREAST: HOT MOMS CLUB BREASTFEEDING FAVORITES

If you are going to breastfeed, do it in style and splurge—you deserve it.

❀ Bébé au Lait (www.bebeaulait.com) has the coolest breastfeeding cover-up (aka Hooter Hiders), ensuring that neither your style nor your modesty will be compromised.

❀ Bella Materna's nursing lounge dress is perfect for afternoons out or just hanging out at home. For the perfect combination of sexiness, functionality, and comfort, check out www.bellamaterna.com.

❀ Chapter 5 has a whole section on finding the perfect nursing bra, with references to all the most popular brands.

BUMP ON A BUDGET

Belly Fish (www.belly-fish.com) is a nursing cover and pillow all in one, priced under $50. They come in stylish colors and designs and are the perfect multifunctional cover.

ECO-MINDED MAMA

Kai Kids (www.kaikids.com) bamboo nursing pads are good for not only the earth but your boobs as well! Eco-friendly, they slip right into your bra, and they are invisible under a snug shirt and superabsorbent, saving you from embarrassing leakage.

Remember you are a Hot Mom and you can handle anyone and anything that comes your way. It's all part of the experience, so do what you feel is right and try to keep your sense of humor!

JOURNAL—MONTH THREE

1. What is the silliest pregnancy advice that has come your way?

_____

_____

_____

_____

_____

_____

_____

_____

_____

_____

2. Your version of your pregnancy story. Here's your big chance all you scribes, poets, songwriters, and even list makers to create the play-by-play of your pregnancy. And you can be as deliberately ridiculous or Pollyanna-ish or plain over-the-top as you like, because we all know every birthing is unique. Get creative. Tap into ancient myths. Use your imagination to conjure up the delivery experience of your dreams!

_____

_____

_____

_____

_____

_____

_____

_____

_____

_____

_____

_____

_____

_____

_____

_____

3. Take time to write out all the good advice from your circle of support. When you're feeling unsure or have a bad day, take this out and remind yourself that you're surrounded by loving people with sound opinions you know you can always count on.

_____

_____

_____

4. What did your Hot Mom-to-be intuition tell you today?

_____
_____
_____
_____
_____
_____
_____
_____

5. Record your most wicked and wild food craving.
    Take a picture for future evidence.

_____
_____
_____
_____
_____
_____
_____
_____
_____
_____
_____

6. What's the craziest thing that makes you cry—
Simon Cowell berating your favorite singer? And
what's making you happy—the color mauve?
Ginger lemon tea? A favorite pair of comfy shoes?

_____

_____

_____

_____

_____

_____

_____

_____

_____

_____

_____

_____

_____

_____

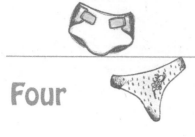

Four

Daddy Gadgetitis

*The difference between men and boys
is the price of their toys.*

—Proverb

Congratulations! If you're like most women, you've just escaped the grip of morning sickness and are entering what's called "The Golden Age of Pregnancy"—the middle trimester, when your body supposedly feels better. But this is still a time of many changes. A lot is happening, and it's hard not to be overwhelmed by all the new events going on in and around you. You're experiencing wild food cravings, along with amazing mood swings—and all the while you're starting to truly feel the presence of your little passenger. Yeah, and sometimes your bodily functions aren't exactly ladylike. Excuse you!

And in a closet somewhere, a bewildering stack of baby items magically starts to accumulate. I can hear you thinking, *Do I really need a baby-bottom fan? Or the Walk-Along-Baby-Hoist?* Furthermore, all this is going on just as childbirth and newborn questions start demanding your answers: What color should you paint the baby's room? Are you going natural or C-section? When do you want the baby shower and who should be on the list? Lamaze, Bradley, or hypnotherapy childbirth? To top it off, your spouse or partner—who is just starting to realize the responsibilities in the months (and years!) to come—may be acting just a little strange!

When it comes down to it, newborns really need only a few things: you (the source of comfort, love, and food), a place to sleep, some soft clothing of various kinds, diapers and diaper gear (changing mat, wipes, etc.), bath accessories, bottles for feeding, and a car carrier. Oh, and if your baby's room is down the hall, a good monitor might be useful, and . . . hmm, let me think . . . um, food and water. Yes, that would be good. For at least the first couple of months, all the other stuff is gravy, since all little one will really be doing is sleeping and pooping a lot.

"Diaper backward spells repaid. Think about it."
—Marshall McLuhan

That's a load of crap!

What Is Your Baby's Carbon Butt Print?

It is amazing that we take the most biodegradable thing on the planet—poop—and wrap it in plastic that takes up to five hundred years to decompose. Americans toss away enough disposable diapers each year to reach the moon and back at least seven times. I admit I used disposable diapers with my son, and when I thought of re-usable diapers at the time, I pictured cloth and pins. But there have been incredible developments in diapers in recent years—the cloth diaper has been reinvented by companies like bumGenius, Happy Heinys, Fuzzi Bunz, Diapers and Bumkins, all of which make cloth diapers that are easily fastened and can be used over one hundred times. Nature Baby Care Diapers are the first eco-friendly disposable diapers. They use natural-based and compostable materials. If you are interested in exploring more eco-friendly alternatives, visit www.diapersetc.com and www.diapers.com.

BUMP ON A BUDGET

Tear wipes in half the long way, down the middle. They will last twice as long, and they are easier to use for little bums and small changes.

ECO-MINDED MAMA

Changing diapers can overpower even the sweetest of baby smells. Squeeze a lemon into your diaper bucket or genie; this is a natural way to neutralize odor rather than using aerosol air fresheners.

Another Kind of "Baby Crap"

Babies may not need that much stuff, but there's a whole world of knickknacks and accessories that can tempt you because they seem so darn cute. Or useful. OR ABSOLUTELY NECESSARY . . . for at least a week or two. For instance, special diaper disposal units sold by the thousands seem to be on the list of "useless items" for many moms afterward. And, surprisingly, separate bottle warmers quickly get sent to the back of the shelf in favor of microwaves and the traditional on-the-stove method. So before you start stocking up, check with friends or with online mom communities about the latest gear. Once you hear the tales of closets full of discarded and unused items, you can simplify and feel assured that more is not necessarily better!

This will also help with registering your needs for a baby shower. Instead of the pack-and-play baby entertainment center that's difficult to carry and impossible to fold, maybe you could list the all-important postpartum mom massage! Or the completely necessary lunch for four at your favorite restaurant. It's good to remind friends (especially the childless ones) that keeping in touch—or at least a bit in touch—with your personal desires will make you a happier mom, friend, and person.

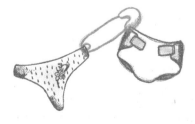

Be Savvy about Baby Stuff

As soon as the ultrasound declares a boy or girl will be arriving, we see visions of pink and blue or yellow and green in our minds. From cradle and crib bedding to the outfit we will dress him or her in the day we leave the hospital, lists immediately start being made and grow longer and longer with everyone else's suggestions. Baby showers are the tip of the iceberg as pregnancy hormones cause us to think everything we scanned for the baby registry isn't enough for our little ones. Waddling into the local baby store, we pull out a cart and purchase last-minute additions we know we will need.

Product manufacturers bank on our ignorance as first-time expectant parents. They know we read every checklist—some of them are even created by juvenile product manufacturers—because the first time around we believe being a good parent includes buying the best, the newest, and the prettiest for our baby. First time around, you wouldn't dare let your baby's bottom go cold, and you think the diaper wipe warmer is needed. Weeks into hearing the baby cry at 3:00 a.m. while you wait for the diaper wipe to warm, you realize your newborn doesn't need it. Same for the amount of blankets you picked up and the number of strollers, carriers, and bouncy seats you just "had to have."

I take care of three little ones now, but I can remember being pregnant the first time. Sure, my first child ended up with a few dozen baby blankets; however, the second time around, I knew what was essential and what definitely wasn't. We were going to be good parents whether our kid's stroller cost $85 or $750. Not having the same pre-walkers as seen on the kid of an A-lister doesn't mean our children will flunk out of kindergarten. I promise. Take it from me, every week I sort through hundreds of baby and children's products sent from companies hoping you'll buy from them. Research and be practical. You too can be a Savvy Mommy.

—Victoria Pericon,
media personality, mom of three,
and founder of *Savvy Mommy* magazine.

"Post-Party Depression" and Other Little-Known Diseases

They say almost 80 percent of all fathers experience some sympathetic pregnancy symptoms. The most common is weight gain. Sympathetic pregnancy, or *couvade,* happens in many forms, with men complaining of indigestion, back pain, even morning sickness. It gets a little tricky when he starts joining you in mood swings. Some women think it's a ploy to get the attention back on the guy's side of the court, but I believe it's more useful to think of it as your partner's way of expressing concern and empathy. Furthermore, why not have a partner in passing gas? Then you have someone else to blame it on! If your man really wants to know what pregnancy feels like, get him a belly suit and check out www.empathybelly.org.

Some men also feel a little at a loss with the rearranging of life and home. Maybe, just maybe, your guy was used to being the center of attention, and, as much as you'd like to say, "Hey, guy, remember who's having the BABY!" there is a change going on for him too. Fathers-to-be have been know to get a bit blue or cranky since you're not going out and doing all the things you used to. I guess you could call it "post-party depression."

But there is a simple solution: like any other communications challenge, find a gentle way to engage him. With a dad, it's good to give him a problem that needs a solution. Enlist him in building something for the baby's room, or if he's into design, give him the color quest for paint and fabric. Ask him to set up a new home music system or to create a better backyard for those more frequent at-home occasions. And—I know it can be difficult—let him take charge.

Also, I'm well aware that sometimes it's the "sports room" or the extra home office that becomes the baby's room. If that's the case, encourage him to claim some space and celebrate his favorite team elsewhere in your home. And if the zippy new car has to wait because of the minivan, let him compensate with a strong case of gadgetitis!

You know the baby's room? No? Oh, you are not familiar with this room? Well, perhaps you'll recognize it by what it is currently known as: your music room. It's the extra room you proclaimed as your own when you moved into your house. It's the room you used to escape to when your wife was watching some bullshit movie on the Lifetime network. . . . Now that room, your sanctuary, is going to be covered in fluffy bunnies and baby accessories. Take down the Budweiser mirror . . . you're being evicted. This may be the first time you realize that not only is the baby consuming all of your thoughts and conversations but it's also taking over your house! And the weirdest part is that the baby isn't even here yet!

—Michael Crider,
author of *The Guy's Guide
to Surviving Pregnancy, Childbirth,
and the First Year of Fatherhood*

Make Room!

You are adding another member to your family. The whole energy in the house is about to change. You may view decorating the baby's room as an exciting adventure or a dreadful task. Transitions are always challenging. No matter what your style, it is important to create a warm, soothing space for the baby, as this will ease the transition for both of you! Use your senses to create a baby sanctuary for sleep.

Your baby's room represents a clean slate, a new beginning. Before decorating, air out the room, open the windows, and—although this may sound a little silly—clap your hands or ring some bells; doing either can also help clear the old energy.

- ✿ *Relaxing sounds.* Think of a ticking clock, a recording of the beach or ocean waves, or even a fan. Anything rhythmic will help lull your little one and remind him of those peaceful days tucked safely inside your womb (www.babymusictogo.com).

- ✿ My friends with babies rave about the award-winning Sleep Sheep (www.sleepsheepandfriends.com). The cuddly sheep has different soothing sounds to ensure a tranquil environment for your baby's sleep; we have gifted many celebrity moms with the Sleep Sheep, and all have been very thankful!

- ✿ *Pleasing smells.* Babies have a strong sense of smell, and nothing smells better to them than YOU! So the week or two before your little one arrives, sleep with her blankets and bedding so the scent will remind your baby of you and help her feel secure.

✿ *Keep things visually simple.* Babies can get overwhelmed with too much stimulation. Bedsheets in a solid color are more pacifying than loud patterns. Painting the walls earth tones is ideal for achieving a mellow, nurturing feeling. www.serenaandlily.com has soft-color paints with low odors that are among the least toxic on the market. Choose all the colors that you like. However, remember it is not safe for pregnant women to inhale the fumes. So while your family or friends do the painting, plan a shopping day, spa day, or trip—enjoy your free time while you can!

Using Feng Shui techniques will help you position the furniture in the baby's room to create an atmosphere that helps comfort and inspire, rather than contributing to poor sleeping habits or crankiness. *A Peaceful Nursery: Preparing a Home for Your Baby with Feng Shui* by Alison Forbes is the perfect guide. A more expensive but custom alternative would be to hire "The Feng Shui Guy" to come and personally arrange your baby's space (www.thefengshuiguy.com).

The award-winning Zaky, an innovative pillow for babies that mimics the loving touch of a mother's hand, is the ideal way for your new baby to feel bonded and protected. Zakys have been especially beneficial with premature or sick babies. Learn more at www.zakeez.com.

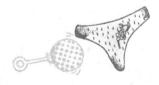

Sit Back and Order Room Service

There are so many great options now for crib and room décor—long gone are the days of cartoon clichés.

> Celebrities today are moving away from themed rooms and more into classic beautiful spaces. I always recommend products and décor that will grow with your child. Opt for a three-in-one crib that will transition into a toddler bed, and invest or splurge on a great rocker or glider; you will be spending a lot of time rocking and feeding the baby, and a nice one will still work in your child's room as a favorite reading chair for you both.
> —Natalie Klein,
> Hot Moms Club celebrity baby planner

Best of all, you don't even have to leave your house to decorate your baby's room completely—talk about room service. There are dozens of great websites with baby furniture and accessories to suit any style.

A few of my favorite nursery decorating spots:

Million Dollar Baby (www.milliondollarbaby.com)
New Arrivals, Inc. (www.newarrivalsinc.com)
The Land of Nod (www.landofnod.com)
Pottery Barn Kids (www.potterybarnkids.com)
Modern Nursery (www.modernnursery.com)
Hip Baby Gear (www.hipbabygear.com)

Restoration Hardware Kids (www.rhbabyandchild.com)
Modern Tots (www.moderntots.com)
Netto Collection (www.nettocollection.com)
Bratt Decor (www.brattdecor.com)
Banana Fish (www.bananafishinc.com)

BUMP ON A BUDGET

One of my favorite baby and home designers, Dwell-Studio (www.dwellshop.com), is now available at Target and more affordable than ever. This is a great way to get that designer look for less.

As an affordable alternative to a mural or painting a wall design, Wall Candy Art (www.wallies.com) peel-and-stick designs allow you to stick on fun wall designs, decals, and murals so they can easily be removed as the child grows. They have some really adorable options under $20.

Check out www.Wonderfulgraffiti.com for custom monograms, sayings, and phrases that stick to and remove easily from your walls. These stick-ons could be your baby's name or initials, or a nursery rhyme or favorite saying. They add a unique and gorgeous touch to any room, starting at $25.

A reasonable way to organize is to use clear plastic bins and containers. They cost under $10 and are perfect for storing clothes that are too big or out of season. Purchase a pack of unlined cardstock and label the bins for size and season. When you are done packing the bins, place the cardstock in the front so you can easily find the size you are looking for when glancing in the closet. Sugar Booger closet dividers are a great way to organize baby clothes that hang in the closet. They offer adorable designs to fit in between hangers with decals so you can label them Newborn, 3-6 months. etc. Packets of five start at $10, and they can be found at www.paisleymonkey.com.

Framing and hanging paintings or drawings from other siblings or nieces and nephews is an inexpensive way to add color, and a personal touch to any nursery.

To get the best bang for your buck, when shopping for a crib, make sure but a 3 in 1, that it converts to a toddler bed. A majority of cribs are built this way today, so there are plenty of stylish options.

$TUFF TO DROOL OVER!

Kidtropolis (www.kidtropolisbuild.com) creates incredible custom-built kid's rooms. These functional and unique one-of-a-kind spaces start in the five figures!

Lulla Smith (www.lullasmith.com)offers a luxury line of baby linens and bassinets fit for a prince or princess. She uses only the finest cottons and silks, and her items can be found in the nurseries of Jennifer Lopez, Tom Cruise and Katie Holmes, Courtney Cox and many other celebrities.

At Muu Furniture (www.muukids.com), featuring upscale modern décor, cribs retail for $1375 and up. The website www.sparkability.net has a huge selection of upscale items for baby nursery and home. You might find Tavo high chairs, which look like expensive bar stools and easily blend with your décor, for $345.

Mod Mama (www.modmama.com) is a luxury modern baby boutique filled high-ticket items to drool over!

Having an artist hand paint a design or mural in the nursery can be gorgeous. If this is something you plan to invest in, be sure to create something that isn't too babyish; your little one will grow fast, and you will be painting over it before you know it. Artist Vanessa Verillion created nontoxic wall sticks in a variety of creative motifs. You can purchase four sheets for $31 at www.mysweetmuffin.com.

ECO-MINDED MAMA

A lot of celebrities today are opting for eco-friendly nurseries. *Ugly Betty* star Ana Ortiz worked with Hot Moms Club to create such a room for her first baby.

If you're looking for companies that are eco-friendly or offer organic options, these are some of the great companies we used in pulling together Ana's nursery.

Giggle (www.giggle.com)
DwellStudio (www.dwellshop.com)
Duckduck (www.duckduck.com) all organic
Oeuf (www.oeufnyc.com)
Bambino Land (www.bambinoland.com)
Baby Earth (www.babyearth.com)
Serena & Lily (www.serenaandlily.com)
Sage Creek Organics (www.sagecreekorganics.com)
The Little Seed (www.thelittleseed.com)
fawn&forest (www.fawnandforest.com)
AFM Safecoat (www.afmsafecoat.com)
The Ultimate Green Store
    (www.theultimategreenstore.com)

Great Green Resources:

Green Nest (www.greennest.com) and Healthy Child Healthy World (www.healthychild.org) both have tips and information on creating a "green" nursery and a healthy toxin-free home environment for you and for the new baby. The blogs Teensygreen (www.teensygreen. com) and Eco Stiletto Kids (www.ecostiletto.com) profile environmentally safe products and give advice for mom and baby.

While you are having fun with the details, don't forget that being organized is one of the more important things you can do to help yourself once the baby arrives. I am sure you are starting to compile an avalanche of baby clothes and things. The Container Store www.container store.com has the solution for all of your organizing needs. They will customize containers to your closet.

If you have other children, let them assist in preparing and decorating the new baby's room. Children tend to be very territorial and often see the baby as an invasion of "their" space. Allowing them to join in creating the space for their new brother or sister helps to give them a sense of control and pride. Letting them choose or arrange the toy area and letting them create artwork for the room is fun for them and also a way to add charm to any baby's room.

It may be premature, but while you are starting to get your house ready for the new arrival, you should also be thinking about babyproofing. Kimberlee Mitchell is a child safety expert and the founder of Boo Boo Busters, she sits on the Hot Moms Club advisory board, and she's the "go-to" guru for celebrity parents who want to childproof their homes. She has Boo Boo Busted the homes of Katie and Tom Cruise, Matt Damon, Britney Spears, and Tom Brady. Most infamously, she spent an entire day at the Octomom's home getting it ready for her brood. If you don't live in California, don't worry: you can still learn from her expertise. She has a great blog filled with tips and ideas. Visit www.boobobusters.com. To find a babyproofing service in your area, go to www. babyproofingdirectory.com for help. Just plug in your zip code, and the site will spit out all of the babyproofing services near you.

While we are talking about safety, now is a great time to brush up on your CPR skills. There are different techniques for babies and toddler emergencies, and the more prepared you are, the more calm and confident you will be if in fact you should ever have to put those skills to the test. Call your local hospital or school and find out when they offer CPR classes or babysitter training courses.

Here are some great references to have around the house or to keep in the car: SafetyMate (www.safetymate. com) is a voice-operated first aid and emergency instruction device. Medbasics (www.babymedbasics.com) is a quick reference guide designed to clip onto your stroller or diaper bag, or fit in your glove compartment. Emergency Café (www.emergencycafe.com) is another good resource. It has several pre-packed emergency backpacks for all situations.

Gadgetitis

Men love their toys. I'll never forget the day my husband came home with a baby video spy camera and mini baby TV monitor. Mind you, the baby's room was right next to our bedroom—if I leaned my head far enough to the right, I could see his crib. My husband spent hours mounting this infrared beam at the foot of the crib, getting the position just right. He had an excited twinkle in his eye, all the while bragging about how we would be able to see the baby's every move in the pitch dark. If the baby burped the wrong way, leaned the wrong way, or twisted or coughed, we would be on the scene and ready to act.

The excited dad-to-be also bought a souped-up baby stroller that had more features and cup holders than my car. If he could have added chrome wheels, I think he would have. Now, I would have preferred something a bit more sedate, but it's also good if dad likes the features of the new "car"; that way he's more encouraged to be part of the walking routine. So bring your hubby with you when you "test drive" strollers; he'll have fun with all of the new models on the market today!

Your stroller may be one of the most important purchases you make, so be sure to do your research. I encourage you to try out different types to see which will fit your lifestyle. Determine what your needs are. Do you like to run or hike? Will you need a stroller that can maneuver on tough terrain? If you live in a city, making sure your stroller can easily fit through doorways and has quick handling functionality would be a priority.

Maybe you need a stroller that will accommodate another child as well, maybe your car is small and you need something lightweight and easy to store and pack. Or maybe you just want to make a statement and look chic when rolling out to the park for playdates. Really think about how you will be using your stroller so you can buy one that best fits your needs. Ask friends how they like the one they have, and get out there and try them out.

There are so many innovative strollers today that the choices are vast and overwhelming. I could write a whole book on strollers and the gadgets that go with them, but here is a quick breakdown of some Hot Moms Club favorites in each category.

Best-Looking or Statement Strollers

Mutsy (www.mutsybaby.com): my favorite for sleek, modern, ultracool design

Quinny Buzz (www.quinny.com): European design, in bright colors with lots of cool accessories

Bugaboo (www.bugaboostrollers.com): known as the Hollywood "it" stroller, offering metallic special collections and versions by designers like Paul Frank and Marc Jacobs

DADS ARE THE NEW MOM

The Rock Star Baby (www.rockstarbaby.com) stroller is all black with embroidered or Swarovski crystal skulls. The line was started by Bon Jovi drummer Tico Torres.

Baby Planet (www.baby-planet.com) offers eco-friendly strollers. They have a variety of innovative designs and double strollers, and are partnered with the Wildlife Conservation Society; you can even have an endangered species line of strollers.

Unique Design

Orbit (www.orbitbaby.com) is the world's first rotating stroller; you can turn the base at any angle.

Stokke Xplory (www.stokkeusa.com) is an upright pram that elevates your child so he or she can be closer to you.

Teutonia (www.teutoniausa.com) personalize your stroller; you can choose the wheels, the patterns, and colors. Fun and sleek!

$TUFF TO DROOL OVER!

The Roddler Custom Stroller starts at $2,500 (www.kidkustoms.com). It has a hot rod look and sleek design. They will custom match the paint to your car and let you choose what material the seats and cover are made from; they offer everything from vegan options to the most premium leathers.

Silver Cross (www.silvercross.co.uk) has been around since 1877. They are known for their elegant prams; their Heritage Collection has a time-honored fashion and look with a modern twist. They start at $1,000.

Favorite Strollers for Jogging

BOB Sport Utility (www.bobgear.com) is the leader and most popular jogger stroller.

Mountain Buggy (www.mountainbuggy.com) has a sleek design and variety of colors.

InStEP (www.instep.net) offers both fixed and swivel wheel models.

Favorite Strollers for Twins

BumblerideIndie Twin (www.bumbleride.com) can easily fit through doorways and has swivel wheels for easy maneuvering.

Maclaren Twin Triumph (www.maclarenbaby.com) isn't the best-looking stroller out there, but when it comes to convenience, this one can't be beat. Along with many other features, its quick five-second, one-hand foldability is a huge selling point to any parent of twins.

Valco Baby Tri Mode Twin (www.valcobaby.com) has an add-on toddler seat so it can comfortably ride three.

Best Tandem to Fit an Older Child

phil&teds inline collection (www.philandteds.com)
Joovy Big Caboose (www.joovy.com)
Peg Perego Duette SW (www.pegperego.com)

Favorite Portable

Maclaren Easy Traveler Stroller's frame fits almost every car seat model. It's easy to fold and store in your car trunk for quick trips.

Mia Moda Facile (www.miamodainc.com) makes a lightweight umbrella stroller that handles well and looks sharp.

BUMP ON A BUDGET

Prince Lionheart stroller connectors (www.princelion heart.com) snap and connect two umbrella strollers so you can walk them side by side together, as if they were one stroller. $13

If you receive a stroller from a relative or want to refresh one from your first child, My Monkey Moo Stroller Pads (www.mymonkeymoo.com) are stylish and fun at $69. The colors and designs will make any stroller look new and exciting again. Sure to turn heads in any playgroup!

Best Stroller for City Moms

Baby Jogger, City Mini (www.babyjogger.com) weighs less than seventeen pounds and was designed with city moms in mind.

StrollAway by Metrotots (www.metrotots.com) is the perfect stroller hook for your stroller. It fits perfectly on the back of your door so that the overpriced but fabulous stroller you just bought fits neatly and won't take up too much of your 1,000-square-foot apartment!

The website www.strollermama.com sells many of the

strollers I mentioned and has video displays of how each one works. It is a great site to reference and use as a resource when finding your "perfect match" in a stroller.

Pimp Your Ride

Many of the stroller companies mentioned above offer cool accessories to customize and upgrade your ride, just like in a car.

Some Hot Moms Club favorites:

Girlie things you'll love

Snuggle Mez (www.snugglemez.com) car seat snugglers and blankets are stylish, cozy, and functional.

blankyclip (www.blankyclip.com) is a cute and safe way to keep your blanket from falling off your stroller.

WooBee, by Rain or Shine Kids (www.rainorshinekids.com), makes supersoft and cozy blankets that tie onto your stroller or car seat, and they are good for any season or any climate.

Gadgety things he'll love

Strollometer Computer (www.rei.com) is a speedometer for your stroller.

Click 'n Go Stroller Accessory System by Prince Lionheart (www.princelionheart.com) fits most strollers. It includes two adjustable clips, a swivel cup holder, snack cup, bottle holders—it holds something for everyone in the family.

Kiddopotamus Piddle Pad (www.kiddopotamus.com) is a waterproof seat liner, and it slips comfortably and discreetly in the stroller or car seat.

Sunshine Kids Stroll-light (www.sunshinekidsbaby.com) strobe light can be easily attached to the back of the stroller to alert cars when walking at dusk.

Protect a Bub sunshades (www.protect-a-bubusa. com) can be used on your stroller and car seats.

Your Other Ride

As your belly expands, you will find it more and more challenging and uncomfortable to drive. Make sure your seat belt tucks BELOW your tummy, not over it. Don't worry about the chest strap—it's fine, but the bottom belt should rest on your hips. There are devices to loosen your belt if it is feeling too tight. The Maternity Seatbelt (www.onestepahead.com) is a great product designed to ensure that your seat belt won't ride up on your belly. Experts advise keeping the air bag on but adjusting your seat so that it remains at least twelve inches from the steering wheel. You should be as far away as you can but still be able to comfortably reach the pedals.

Rock That Minivan!

If you think you can kiss any leftover sex appeal good-bye the minute you trade in your Miata for a minivan, think again. Minivans have come a long way, and after you realize what a pain in the butt it is to pack the stroller and all the baby gear into your sedan, it won't be long before you'll be shopping for a bigger vehicle. For some, this can be traumatic at first (one comedian compared the experience to a dog getting neutered), so ease into it. When my son was young, I had an SUV, and with all his gear, it still felt small at times! Today I have a sportier car. After a minor fender bender, it had to spend a week in the repair shop, so the rental place offered me a minivan until a more desirable car became available. I admit I was mortified; I would park far away from my meetings so no one would see me getting in or out. My son, on the other hand, thought it was the greatest thing that he could sit in the third row. He raved about it and begged me to keep it. Bottom line, you may lose a few "cool" points for owning one, but if you have a few kids or a busy schedule and a baby you will love the convenience. Remember, that third row pulls down (wink wink), so if you have to or choose to get yourself a minivan, don't forget to make it rock now and then—literally!

The "Dad" Factor

I must say that even since the time I had my son, the "dad factor" has become much more visible. It's common to see men with strollers or baby backpacks going for a walk or heading to the park . . . and it's not considered unmanly. It's all part of sharing the parenting, which is more popular now than it was just ten years ago.

Consider yourself lucky! Companies are even offering diaper bags and products tailored for dads.

A perfect place to give in to gadgetitis is at DadGear (www.dadgear.com). The site has the most innovative diaper bag/diaper vest/jackets on the market. With practical compartments and cool designs, your guy can help without losing an ounce of his manhood. Diaper Dude (www. diaperdude.com) has a wide selection of diaper bags for dad with camo, skulls, and other manly colors and designs. And what man can resist waiting for a newborn with *The Godfather* DVD giving him fatherly advice in a godfatherly way? Another fun site is Baby Wit (www.babywit.com), which has shirts for babies with silly sayings like *I'm already smarter than the president,* and funny ones for dad that say, *I was here first!* And finally, you've got to check out Baby Gizmo's site: www.babygizmo.com.

> "Any man can be a father, but it takes a special man to be a dad."
> —Unknown

Your guy will love this!

Combi has an iPod bouncer, which allows you to plug in your iPod to the baby bouncer seat and play your own music so you don't have to listen to another annoying version of "Twinkle Twinkle Little Star" over and over again. Now you can stream Enya or U2 or another of your relaxing favorites so baby can snooze and you can relax too ($80 at www.thinkgeek.com).

We all know how important it is to capture on film the birth and all of the precious baby moments afterwards. Flip Video Ultra (www.theflip.com) is small, convenient, and plugs easily into your computer so you can email footage to relatives and friends. It's offered in fun colors and costs under $150. Upgrade to the Flip Mino in HD. It's the world smallest HD camcorder and costs under $230.

TOP DAD BLOG SITES

Being Dad (www.beingdadusa.com)
Dad Gone Mad (www.dadgonemad.com)
The Goodfather (www.drmoz.com)
The Family Man (www.familymanonline.com)
DadLabs, for guys with "Daditude" (www.dadlabs.com)

BEST BOOKS TO GET HIM

The Guy's Guide to Surviving Pregnancy,
    Childbirth, and the First Year of Fatherhood
    by Michael Crider
My Boys Can Swim! by Ian Davis
Mack Daddy by Larry Bleidner
Be Prepared; A Practical Handbook for New
    Dads by Gary Greenberg and Jeanine Hayden

If your man is more comfortable riding a Harlem subway at night than holding a newborn, Boot Camp for New Dads (www. daddybootcamp.org) is perfect for him. Available in over thirty-five states, these classes are intense training for dads to learn how to care for their little angels.

<u>Diaper Bag Envy</u>

Diaper bags have come a long way since I was pregnant. The choice of bags then consisted of Winnie the Pooh or plaid. Today the functionality is outstanding, and there are endless choices to fit any style. Like your purse, your diaper bag will be your biggest accessory, literally attached to your hip for the next year of your life. So do yourself a favor: invest in one you really love—or throw it on your baby shower registry!

Here are my favorites in every price range:

Munchkin Jelly Bean Cargo Sling ($28) is a diaper bag and baby cargo carrier all in one. If you are an active mom, this is the perfect accessory. While you still need a traditional diaper bag, this is the perfect easy tote for baby and your stuff on trips to the zoo, the beach, or other outings.

As a brand, *Skip Hop* ($29 to $90) has mastered

functionality and style, and their diaper bags are no exception. Their collection is affordable and head turning (www.skiphop.com).

Dante Beatrix bags ($36 to $220) are the ultimate stroller accessory! They have special clips that fasten to the stroller and extend to carry across your body (www.dantebeatrix.com).

From *Reese Li,* the Fairfax Changing Clutch ($60 to $150) holds three to five diapers and is perfect to attach to your stroller for quick changes (www.reeseli.com).

Original Diaper Dude for the Diva ($65 to $99) offers an original hands-free, compact diaper bag (think fanny pack but cool) in canvas or faux patent leather (www.diaperdude.com).

The website www.oioi.com.au offers a huge selection of fun styles to fit any taste, from the sporty to the girly-girl. Check out the *OiOi* ($100 to $130).

From *Ju-Ju-Be,* the Be Prepared bag ($150 to $200) is perfect for mothers expecting twins. It has color-coded tabs to remind you what pocket is for which child, crumb drains, and more. This bag gives you everything but the kitchen sink (www.ju-ju-be.com).

Petunia Pickle Bottom ($175–$350). A staple among Hollywood moms, including Alison Sweeney, Petunia is known for her classic feminine styles. Their Cross Town Clutch has a fold-out changing pad and room for a diaper and wipes (www.petuniapicklebottom.com).

From *Maelee Baby,* the Chloe Bag ($225) has the softest leather. Available in black, brown and white leather, stylish and subtle, you would never guess it's a diaper bag (www.maeleebaby.com).

Kate Spade Baby Bags ($235 to $525) offer the classic Kate Spade look with diaper bag functionality and changing pads included (www.katespade.com).

Mia Bossi's bag ($350 to $450) is so stylish that you'll want to use it long after the little one is out of diapers. Katie Holmes and other celeb moms have been known to sport them (www.miabossi.com).

A favorite among celebrity moms like Angelina Jolie, *Suzy Diaper Bag by Hammitt* ($595) is the ultimate splurge (www.hammittbags.com).

Design Your Own bag! If you would like to create or design your own custom diaper bag, visit *B's purses* at www.bspurses.com. You can choose the lining, fabric, hardware, and handle. Browse dozens of styles and colors to suit any taste.

Goober Baby has gift sets of coordinating changing mats, changing purses, and holders for all of baby's supplies in adorable designs. They fit nicely into any bag, or use on their own (www.gooberbaby.com).

BUMP ON A BUDGET

JJ Cole's Carry All Tote (JJ Cole, $19 to $69) is by far the coolest diaper bag on the market under $20. Also, their Tactic Changing purse is in a sense a diaper clutch. These are the best bags for the buck (www.jjcoleusa.com). The Kemby Sidekick (Kemby, $168) is a diaper bag AND baby carrier all in one. Use the diaper bag on its own or quickly transform it into a convenient baby carrier. The Kemby Sidekick has won several innovation awards and is the ultimate two-for-one (www.kemby.com).

ECO-MINDED MAMA

Fleurville bags ($69 to $150) come with a unique polyurethane exterior that resists cracking, abrasions, temperature changes, and spills. Fleurville offers a wide variety of styles and is a completely green company, using eco-friendly materials, as well as business practices (www.fleurville.com). Go GaGa Slide Tote Bag ($128) is perfect for moms or dads; its patented ergonomic strap distributes the weight of the bag across your back. It comes with a changing pad and a strap to hold your yoga mat (www.gogagalife.com).

$TUFF TO DROOL OVER!

Designer Rebecca Minkoff (www.rebeccaminkoff.com) now offers a signature "Knocked Up" leather bag in several trendy colors ($695). Hush A Bye Baby's (www.hushabyebabyproducts.com) three-in-one diaper bag ($495) is the ultimate in luxury. The material is cotton chenille that is soft and plush, and the bag is cozy and functional. The Louis Vuitton Monogram Mini Lin Diaper Bag for $2,200 is the ultimate splurge.

DADS ARE THE NEW MOM

Here are our favorite diaper bags for your dude. Just like there are for Mom, there are plenty of diaper bags out there to match your man's personality!

Dad Gear (www.dadgear.com) has cool bags that
you can customize with your guy's favorite

college sports team, and cool fleeces with compartments to fit diapers, wipes, and a bottle. This company offers something for every type of dad. Their one-of-a-kind options are perfect for dads with an alternative style, and the diaper fleece jacket is ideal for outdoor enthusiasts or dads who like "cool" things ($80 to $100). *All bags are set up to put in a quick access wipe case.

Diaper Dude (www.diaperdude.com) has a great selection of diaper bags in camoflauge, masculine colors, skulls, etc. Prices range from $60 to $100.

Goober Baby (www.gooberbaby.com) has a Gents Line with a preppy thick corduroy diaper clutch for guys who might not want to carry a "bag" ($28).

Stork Tools by Dr. Moz (www.drmoz.com) is big and sturdy; think briefcase for the rugged (under $50).

BUMP ON A BUDGET—FOR HIM

The Logic Bag by JJ Cole: think fanny pack meets superhero belt. It slings over your shoulder, is durable and the ultimate in practical, and it provides hands-free perfection for any outing—just sling it on your shoulder and go ($30, at wwwjjcoleusa.com).

ECO-MINDED MAN

Diaper Dude has an eco-friendly messenger bag—GREEN DUDE—with the same functionality and style you can expect from the brand but made from recycled PET (plastic water bottles) ($98, at www.diaperdude.com).

Fleurville's DJ BAG is seriously stylish, with superior organization, not to mention the fact that it's environmently friendly. Two thumbs up ($118, at www.fleurville.com).

Passchal offers Dad's Baby Case. Its black eco-friendly leather is made from tractor inner tubes. It looks stunning and can easily double as a briefcase, and each one is unique ($250, at www.passchal.com).

STUFF FOR HIM TO DROOL OVER!

The Petunia Pickle Bottom Scout messenger tote for him in black and brown leather is both gorgeous and functional, the ultimate city or "man bag" ($235, at www.petuniapicklebottom.com).

Stork Sac offers a unisex sac. It's made from pebble cowhide leather, and it's both masculine and stylish, designed to fit not only bottles and baby gear but also a laptop. ($210, at www.storksac.com).

JOURNAL—MONTH FOUR

1. Make a list of your favorite calming music. Make
    sure your CD player or MP3 player is stocked up!

_____

_____

_____

_____

_____

_____

_____

_____

_____

_____

_____

_____

_____

_____

_____

_____

_____

2. Describe your man's response to the upcoming addition to your lives. Denial? Gagetitis? Absolute love and support? (You are lucky!)

_____

_____

_____

_____

_____

_____

_____

_____

_____

_____

_____

_____

_____

_____

_____

_____

_____

_____

3. What baby products are you most excited about purchasing?

_____

_____

_____

_____

_____

_____

_____

_____

_____

_____

_____

_____

_____

_____

_____

_____

_____

_____

_____

_____

4. How are you decorating your nursery?

_____
_____
_____
_____
_____
_____
_____
_____
_____
_____
_____
_____
_____
_____
_____
_____
_____
_____
_____
_____

Five

Bump da Bump, Bump, Bump

I answered the phone one night to a crank call:
"What are you wearing?" he said. I said,
"My MATERNITY UNDERWEAR!" He hung up.
I called back and got his machine.
—Stephanie Blum, comedian, mom of three, and Hot Moms Club Member

Fashion Purgatory

You have passed the in-between period when you don't really look pregnant—just like you ate a couple of Thanksgiving dinners—and now you've officially got the "bump." You may be even starting to think about the bump as a person—with a name, gender, and personality! And with this bump comes the amazing realization, a phrase you've said many times before but now is absolutely 100 percent true: "I have nothing to wear. Really . . . I have NOTHING to wear."

Shopping It Out

Pregnancy is probably the greatest shopping excuse ever! You are actually obligated to shop. Let the fun begin! In the last five years, the phrase *maternity clothes* has taken on a whole new meaning!

Pregnancy clothes have never been more stylish or hip. I was passing a boutique the other day and spotted some cute things in the window. I walked in and was actually about to buy a shirt before I realized it was a maternity store! You no longer have to sacrifice your style or sense of self because you are pregnant. It's so exciting that the trend today is to accentuate that belly, rather than cover it up.

With tummy tats and belly paints, your little embryo can make the best-dressed list before he even leaves the womb! So have fun and go for it.

"Thinking sexy, not size, is the first step to looking sexy," says fashion icon Rebecca Matthias. Founder of Mother's Work Inc., Rebecca Matthias is without a doubt the pioneer of maternity fashion. Mothers Work brands include A Pea in the Pod, Mimi Maternity, Motherhood Maternity, and Destination Maternity. Rebecca dresses more than 2.8 million pregnant moms worldwide each year. And luckily for us, she's willing to share her tips on how easy it is to stay a Hot Mom throughout your pregnancy and beyond.

"The last thing you should do is grab your husband's shirts or sweats for nine months," Rebecca advises. "How you look and how you feel are wrapped together. How you look is a reflection of how you feel, and with so many great maternity fashion options, there is no reason that you can't present yourself to the world with grace and style. If you look good, you'll feel good, and your baby will be happy. It's that simple."

These are Rebecca's five essentials that every pregnant Hot Mom-to-be must have:

1. *It's all in the genes.* Start with a good pair of great preggo jeans. Jeans fit everyone's wardrobe: they can be casual or, with the right top and accessories, flirty and fun. And you don't have to give up your favorite designer fashions—many have pregnancy variations.

2. *Tons of sexy Ts.* Grab an armload of nine-dollar T-shirts in every color—just make sure they have your most flattering neckline. There's no need for a T-shirt to make you look like you're ready for afternoon baseball. Motherhood Maternity has affordable basics that are colorful and easily dressed up with accessories.

3. *Basic black gets your back—and front.* Black pants and/or skirts always do the trick. Think of either of these options as your basic bottom that can anchor every top you can wear. You can create five different looks depending on what you pair your basic black bottoms with: morning coffee, business, afternoon chic, nighttime sexy, and funky.

4. *The secret underneath: sexy lingerie.* Innerwear is the basis of outerwear beauty. You'll know

you look great underneath with beautiful new support and foundation garments that also have a bit of color and lace. There are some great brands of lingerie that are not only comfortable and functional but also allow you to feel sexy. And, yes, thongs have made it to maternity!!

5. *Dress it up.* Dresses are back, any time of year. Summertime dresses are a fun, sexy pregnancy solution, keeping you cool while adding some fashion flair. And in the winter, go long-sleeved and layered for movement and comfort with a stylish look.

Calling Sports Illustrated . . . and Vanity Fair

You may not think so, but pregnancy may be the easiest time of your life to wear a bathing suit. You don't have to have a waist, and the curves are the point! There are great one-pieces, but also consider a tankini two-piece—be daring and show a bit of the belly! Also, sarongs are handy as a cover-up to go from beach to shopping.

And don't hesitate to bring on the bling. Jewelry is also a great friend when the balance of your body shifts. As I said earlier, it is more acceptable now to emphasize the bump. But don't stop there—given the glow on your face and the great hair, why not accessorize with your favorite necklaces and earrings? Be the diva/princess with flair.

Necklaces always fit, so if your fingers are swollen and you have to remove your wedding ring, put it on a chain and wear it around your neck. If it's too scary to have your bling loosely dangling, the Waiting Band is a great alternative. It's an open-ended silver band designed for those days when puffy fingers prevail. They come with special messages, or you can have yours personally engraved (www.tiny-baubles.com).

Rebecca insists that there is only one style no-no in pregnancy: to *not* continue to dress your style. There is no wrong if you continue to express your fashion sense, reinforcing your belief in your instincts, individual beauty, and joy. Don't let anyone tell you that you have to change because you are pregnant!

Beach Bump

Maternity swimsuits are sure to make heads turn. Yeah, I said it, and I mean it!

In my opinion, Prego has the best classic maternity swimsuits, found at www.bellydancematernity.com. Maternal America (www.maternalamerica.com) has my favorite hip, trendy, and very chic maternity bikinis and cover-ups.

There are so many online stores in which to shop for maternity clothing and swimsuits that you could spend hours on the web. I couldn't possibly list all the brands individually, but www.duematernity, www.blossommaternity.com, and www.sierramaternity.com are a few websites that have a variety of pregnancy bathing suites, tankinis, baby-doll beach dresses and all other pregnancy clothing. Old Navy Maternity (www.oldnavy.com) has tankinis and swimsuits for $30 and under.

Destination Maternity stores nationwide are a one-stop shop, with dresses and clothes in every price range. They have an area in which kids can play and men can watch TV, and they also have pregnancy spas, classes, and informational seminars. Visit the website www.destinationmaternity.com and find a location near you.

Maggie Maternity (www.maggiematernity.com) is known for effortless style and comfort. Maggie has created box sets to fit every stage of pregnancy. The Classic Maggie Box contains four essential black pieces. Her Fourth Trimester Maggie Box has four pieces of perfect transition clothes that are comfortable and versatile.

More proof that pregnancy is HOT, and that fashions have come a long way, is the fact that many established designers and celebrities are creating maternity collections. Even Michael Stars and Juicy Couture have a line of maternity shirts and dresses, making it easier than ever to carry your pre-baby style throughout the pregnancy. Nicole Richie launched a Bohemian-chic pregnancy line called "Nicole" for A Pea in the Pod. And *Project Runway* winner Christian Siriano created "Fierce Mamas" maternity line for Moody Mamas (www.moodymamas.com).

$TUFF TO DROOL OVER!

Liz Lange Maternity represents high-end elegance and sophistication. Her stunning collection can be found at www.lizlange.com.

Walking into Rosie Pope's Soho boutique feels like an elegant shop in Paris. The clothes are so stunning that you can hardly believe they are maternity. In addition, she custom makes dresses for all occasions, especially formal ones! Visit www.rosiepope.com.

Isabella Oliver's collection has the most incredible coats and jackets, as well as professional suiting. Take a look at www.isabellaoliver.com.

Vince, Velvet, Hanky Panky, and Diane Von Furstenberg are just a few established brands that have created collections for A Pea in the Pod (www.apeainthepod.com).

And of course your favorite designer jeans like Joe's, 7 for All Mankind, Lucky, True Religion, and many more can be found with a built-in belly band at A Pea in the Pod stores, ranging from $118 to $295.

Hot Moms Club recommends the book *Bump It Up: Transforming Your Pregnancy Poundage Into the Ultimate Style Statement* by Amy Koch to help you navigate all of the fashion possibilities. I got an advance copy of this book, it's great.

BUMP ON A BUDGET

If shelling out a few hundred dollars to buy a pair of your favorite designer jeans is out of reach, try a Belly Belt (www.belly-belt.com) or B-buckles (www.mybbuckles. com). These help expand your favorite pants or jeans. The Bella Band by Ingrid & Isabel (www.ingridandisabel. com) is a favorite among our pregnant moms for making their jeans wearable throughout their pregnancy. None of the products mentioned cost over $30.

Maternity Belly Bands (www.babybeminematernity.

com) are perfect to wear under your T-shirt. They cover your belly and look stylish under cardigans, tanks or tees that were in your pre-baby wardrobe. They're sold in neutral colors or fun prints for $21.99.

Bisou Bisou debuted their maternity collection in JC Penny with a variety of stylish tops and dresses under $40.

Liz Lange for Target (www.target.com) has Liz's sense of style but at a fraction of the cost. I have found dresses in her collection on sale for $15!

Motherhood Maternity (www.motherhood.com) has affordable yet adorable options under $30. Their line of Plus Size Maternity is amazing and affordable also!

Buddha Belly Maternity (www.buddhabellymaternity. com) is young, colorful, and very affordable.

ECO-MINDED MAMA

Maternique (www.maternique.com) offers a selection of eco-friendly pregnancy outfits. Even the packing is made from recycled materials. We love the maternity mini wrap—a three-in-one skirt, top, and hoodie.

Maternity Belly Bands (www.babybeminematernity. com) are also offered in bamboo fabrics.

Expecting Models

Liza Elliott-Ramirez was a professional model in New York for over fifteen years. After becoming pregnant she was surprised that she continued to work extensively, in fact more consistently than any other time in her career.

Seeing the niche, she founded Expecting Models, the first and only agency that specialized in pregnant models. They handle traditional maternity accounts like A Pea in the Pod and Liz Lange, but also American Express, The Olive Garden, and Verizon. One of her models says, "Ten years ago pregnant models really didn't exist—people didn't consider pregnancy as beautiful as they do today." If you are interested in learning more about maternity modeling visit www.expectingmodels.com.

Maternity Bride

Hey, it happens. The website www.maternitybride.com is an incredible venue offering a variety of wedding options for all stages of your pregnancy. You can design the fabric, shades, and styles, and they offer eco-friendly options as well. They also offer custom-designed evening dresses and bridesmaid dresses so you can choose your color and materials.

Momedy

For those with a sense of humor, this is such a fun time to indulge. There are some hilarious shirts out there. These are my favorites:

2 Chix (www.2chix.com) has cute sayings like *You had me at epidural* and *Pregnant is the new sexy.*

Bump—Baby Under Manufacturing Process (www.bumpbabies.com)—offers organic shirts and Sympathy [Bump] shirts for Daddy. I love *Without me there would be no [BUMP]*.

Evil Genius Woman (www.evilgeniuswoman.com) has snarky shirts with attitude like *No touchie*, or *I may be huge, but at least I don't say stupid things to pregnant women*, or *Pregnancy glow my ass, I'm just trying not to hurl*.

Hot Moms Club tees (www.hotmomsclub.com) always get a reaction. We have fun shirts for Dad, Mom, and baby.

Rocker Moms, Not Soccer Moms

For moms with a little edge, Rock Star Moms (www.rockstarmoms.com) has a cool selection of concert maternity tops, from vintage Jimi Hendrix and Rolling Stones to Bon Jovi and Guns N' Roses. They also carry skull tunics, Grateful Dead nursing ponchos, and Run DMC diaper bags. I can't forget the styled NFL pregnancy shirts.

Childish Maternity (www.childishclothing.com and www.Babiesnbellies.com) also has hip clothes for the mom-to-be with a wild side.

Bump on the Go

For those who like to work out, there are tons of great and comfy yoga pants out there, as well as many sites and stores that cater to the mama-to-be who likes to exercise. Fit Maternity (www.fitmaternity.com) has all the clothes you'll need for hiking or the gym. Ocean and Lily (www.maternityactivewear.com) has active wear to get you through all nine months.

For the Bump on Your Bump

You may have noticed that your cute little "innie" belly button is now an "outie" that protrudes from all of your tops, no matter how many layers you're wearing. I happen to think it's sexy and cute when I see a mom-to-be's belly button poke out from her shirt, but I know many women who feel self-conscious about it. If that's the case for you, Miss Oops Popper Stopper (www.mis soops.com) is the solution. Thin and disposable, they cover your belly button pop perfectly. The nonadhesive strip in the center prevents irritation and, yes, they are medically approved!

Lo Beams Nipple and Belly Button Concealers can be found at www.9monthstogrow.com.

Piercings During Pregnancy

Now, it should be said that I don't speak from experience about this topic, but I have done my research and spoken with doctors and a variety of moms who have piercings in all sorts of areas . . . and here is the run-down of what I found. As always, you should refer any specific questions to your physician.

Getting piercings *while* pregnant is not a good idea—not one of the doctors I spoke to approved of getting piercings during maternity in any area, even your ears, as it puts you at unnecessary risk for infections. Getting a naval piercing during maternity was discouraged because your stomach is expanding and changing so much that the hole will have trouble closing properly and leave you again susceptible for an infection, not to mention extra pain and discomfort. If you have had your naval piercing for years before you got pregnant and are wondering whether or not you should remove it, talk to your doctor. Most women I spoke to took it out around five months when it started rubbing against their clothes or stretching too much. Pregnancy Piercings (www.pregnancypiercings.com) offers flexible temporary rings that expand with your belly and are comfortable to wear the entire time. Keep in mind, having a belly button ring generally doesn't affect the birth, and C-section incisions run along the bikini line.

Doctors give less flexibility when it comes to nipple rings. They recommend taking them out right away, especially if you think you will breastfeed. Nipple rings interfere with breastfeeding; they pose a choking hazard to the infant and make it difficult for the baby to latch on properly. Taking the piercing out right away gives the hole a chance to heal, which will help prevent milk from leaking through.

Genital piercings can stay in as long as they are comfortable. It is recommended that you take them out a week or so before labor, due to all the pushing and straining and uncertainty during birth, when they might get ripped out (like your vagina needs any more trauma or discomfort). Better safe than sorry, but talk to your ob-gyn to be sure.

Booby Trap . . .
<u>Taming Those Pregnancy "Perks"!</u>

I waited my whole life to have big boobs, and when I was pregnant I certainly got them in spades. I was so excited to walk into Victoria's Secret and finally purchase something that had less padding then Tom Brady's uniform. Trying on lacy bra after sexy lacy bra, I was thrilled at how my new *hoo-has* looked, but it didn't take long after I got home to realize that more came with big breasts then nice cleavage. My back was hurting and the underwire was digging into my skin, and I was worried all the time about leaking through my shirt. I thought, *Beauty is pain, right?* Well, not for me: I was back at the store in no time, returning my sexy bras and exchanging them for comfy, *padded* maternity ones, a mirror of my old bras—just *bigger.*

That was ten years ago. No one told me to buy a few extra bras in larger cup sizes for after the baby was born, and no one told me that I would be so tired that schlepping to the mall to try on bras after the birth would feel like some kind of cruel torture. I am telling you now, so listen up: getting supportive bras DURING your pregnancy for the time being and beyond is a MUST! Do your research, try on various types and find the best ones for your figure and size. You'll be thanking me afterwards.

Maternity bras are specifically designed without restrictive boning. They often double as nursing bras and are made from softer, more absorbent materials—think leakage, ladies. They're also constructed with special stretch fabrics to accommodate the fact that you may go to sleep with one cup size and wake up with a completely new one in the morning.

Luckily for you, today there are so many advancements in bras—in look, feel, and functionality—that getting a maternity and breastfeeding bra can actually be quite fun. There are even specialists who will help you find your size online and in most maternity stores.

Simply the Breast!

For comfort, style and sex appeal, Condessa (www. condessainc.com), Hot Milk (www.hotmilklingerie. com), Belabumbum (www.belabumbum.com), Bravado (www.bravadodesigns.com), and Eve Alexander (www.evealexander.com) are all great options to help you look like a gorgeous model. *Or you can just wear a bra designed by a gorgeous model:* supermodel Elle Macpherson has a HOT nursing bra in her collection.

For those moms who enjoy more traditional comfort in a bra, Melinda G (www.melindag.com) and Anita (www.anita.com) are great solutions that are still trendy and fun. In addition to supplies and pumps, Medela (www.medelabreastfeedingus.com) has a line of practical breastfeeding bras as well.

BUMP ON A BUDGET

La Leche League (www.llliclothes.com) has a brilliant Wrap 'n Snap bra. It's supercute and priced under $20. It adjusts on the bottom as your bust grows, so it will follow you through all stages and cup sizes and back again. You can wear it comfortably through maternity and nursing and beyond (when your bust goes back to its pre-baby size).

ECO-MINDED MAMA

Bravado (www.bravadodesigns.com) offers green, sustainable fashion nursing bras and clothing. The company also operates in a completely eco-friendly manner. You can read on their website all the ways the company works to preserve the earth. Love it!

Nummies (www.nummies.com) offers a great organic cotton nursing bra.

$TUFF TO DROOL OVER!

Agent Provocateur maternity lingerie collection (www.agentprovocateur.com) is ga-ga gorgeous. Bras are $110 each, and matching panties are $85 a piece.

Finding the Right Bra
for Pregnancy and Breastfeeding

If you're like most women, your breasts were the first clue that you might be expecting. Nipple soreness and breast growth are usually the very first signs of pregnancy. The hormones that are secreted even early on in your pregnancy are already starting to prepare you to be able to feed your baby once it is born. Your body is choosing to breastfeed whether you are or not.

Some women find this perk (no pun intended!) one of the best parts of their new pregnancy body, while others are wondering if their breasts are ever going to stop growing. Regardless of the amount of breast growth you experience during pregnancy, you will be able to make milk and nourish your baby.

Most of this breast growth will occur in the first trimester (up to twelve weeks), but some moms will continue to have growth up until twenty weeks. After twenty weeks, all that is really growing is your rib cage from your belly expanding!

Most advice you read will encourage you to wait until the very end of pregnancy or even after delivery to get your nursing bras. This is usually too late. Trust me—the last thing you will want to do the first week home with your newborn and your engorged leaking breasts is to try on bras! Remember, whether you decide to breastfeed or not, your milk is coming in and you will need these bras for engorgement.

The most important time in a woman's life to have a properly fit bra is during pregnancy and nursing. Some statistics say that up to 90 percent of all women are wearing the wrong size bra!!

First, there are ligaments in your chest wall that support your breasts. When your breasts are bigger and heavier than ever, those ligaments will stretch without the proper support. You may not notice the stretch, because while you are pregnant and nursing, your breasts look good no matter what you do! It's not until after it's all done that you will notice the damage! This is one thing not to skimp on! Either find a place that specializes in fitting bras for pregnancy and breastfeeding, or schedule a virtual consultation. It will be worth the investment. Plastic surgery will cost you much more down the road!

Lastly and most importantly, wearing the wrong size bra or wired bras while breastfeeding can put pressure on the breast tissue and cause problems such as plugged ducts and mastitis (a breast infection). There are many extremely supportive (and even sexy) bras on the market, and with the right fit you will never want to go back to your underwire bras again!

—Shari Criso,
lactation specialist and founder of the
Birth Boutique (www.birthboutique.com)

The Baby Behind the Bump

There's a lot of curiosity right now about just exactly who is developing inside the bump—what little personality, what special look, and, of course, what gender! You may want to be surprised at delivery, to experience that magic moment of seeing your child for the first time and hearing the doctor say, "It's a girl!" or "You've got yourself a little man." I remember that from movies.

But you may want to know. As soon as possible. You may be motivated to find out because you want to bond deeper with your child. Or you may want a head start on names. Or you may want to find out simply because you can start wallpapering in the appropriate pink or blue. Of course, you may just be unable to hold your curiosity for nine months. Whatever your choice, make sure it is what you want to do. Find out, don't find out . . . either way, stand firm. Don't let anyone judge you on your decision. This is your pregnancy, and it doesn't matter if your sister waited or if your best friend consulted every psychic in a ten-mile radius even before she was pregnant.

The decision to find out the sex of your little passenger, your copilot on this crazy ride of pregnancy, is a personal one. My husband and I were anxiously counting down the days to the ultrasound. The need for confirmation of my instincts consumed me. I was so certain it was a boy that the feeling overwhelmed me. Psychologically I was bonding myself with my "little man." If it wasn't a boy, I needed to know as quickly as possible so I could switch gears. I'm sure I could have easily shifted my mind-set to "my girl" at that early stage—really, either gender would have been fine. But I was just dying to know who was inhabiting my belly.

I can remember the day very clearly—the minute the nurse said, "Boy," my husband started howling and jumping around, throwing in dance moves for special effect. It was as if he had scored the winning touchdown in the Super Bowl. He took his enthusiasm out into the hall, hugging anyone he could find (I wish I were exaggerating). He came back into the room and proceeded to call his brother—no answer. His mom—no answer. His dad—no answer. My parents—no. His friend Jon—again, NO ANSWER. He was dying to tell someone, and no one was picking up! As I was getting dressed, I heard him telling someone all the details. "Can you believe that, Pauly? A boy!" Who was Pauly? Pauly? The only Pauly we knew was our mechanic! Yes, the guy that changed our muffler and buffed the dents out of our car was the first person besides us to know the sex of our child.

IntelliGender

If you just can't wait for the sonogram, there is a product called IntelliGender (www.intelligender.com). It claims, via a urine test at as little as six weeks, to be able to determine the sex of the baby. It is sold in drugstores and supermarkets, and although it was correct for the pregnant woman on our team, IntelliGender admits a 10-20 percent chance of error. So take it for fun if you are just too curious to wait.

With both my pregnancies, we did not find out the sex of the baby and have no regrets! Of course, everyone thought we were crazy, and my friends were quite annoyed. But, frankly, I feel like everything in our lives now is so over-communicated, reconfirmed, and just over-planned. Of course I like the world that way (getting an automatic e-mail notification when you place an online order, then when it's shipped, then when it arrives, etc.), but with this special treat . . . it's different. Not knowing the sex allowed my mind to imagine the whole nine months and not form preconceived notions in my head about just exactly what this child would be, would look like, etc. The mystery of it all was almost romantic and thrilling. Yes, I was able to get a nursery done (and very stylishly, of course), and clothes were purchased. Yes, life went on! When my daughter was born, actually they didn't tell us right away what the sex was—I think because they're not used to having to call out, "It's a boy!" or "It's a girl!" anymore! So I was peering up from the other end of the bed when the baby was born, and I saw some round objects between the baby's legs and I said, "Oh, it's a boy!"—but that was just the umbilical cord. They said, "No, it's a girl!" and I was so excited!

—Kristin Moss,
mom of two and
Hot Moms Club member

When I was pregnant, my husband and I had our doctor write the gender of our second child on a slip of paper and put it in a sealed envelope that we brought to dinner with the family. Everyone guessed and elaborated . . . "I think it is a boy, and I will take him to sporting events," and "I think you'll have two girls who will be fabulous sisters." We discussed the possibilities all through dinner. Just before dessert, I opened and read the doctor's note—"I am a girl!" We all screamed and reacted so loudly that other patrons came over to see what all the commotion was! The best thing was that it involved the whole family and gave us a wonderful memory!

—Hilary J. Probst,
teacher, mom of two,
and Hot Moms Club member

We asked the doctor not to tell us the sex of the baby but instead to write it on a card and seal it in an envelope. We planned out an incredibly romantic evening and opened the card together privately. It was wonderful and a beautiful way to learn that we were having a boy—Stefan.

—Katy Wallin-Sandalis,
producer, mom,
and Hot Moms Club member

Step Away from the Bump . . .

Now that you are showing, you may notice that people rub, touch, and lunge for your belly unannounced. I can hardly blame them! Pregnant women are just so darn adorable, ranking right up there with kittens and kiddos. I have to admit that when I see a pregnant woman I know, I just want to touch her tummy like I want to squeeze a cute kid with big cheeks. BUT I remember how uncomfortable it made me when strangers, acquaintances, and friends would grope and grab my belly—and I'm a person who would rather hug than shake hands. Hopefully the horrified look on your face will scare them away, but if it doesn't and you are more reserved than I am, I suggest you get yourself a *Hands off the Belly* T-shirt. You should also get a good defense plan in motion. Although they should, most people won't ask—they will just go for it.

What's in a Name?

How do you choose a name for a child you haven't met? This may be the easiest and most fun part of your pregnancy. (Every doll you had since you were a little girl was named Jill, and, darn it, your baby will be Jill too!) Or it may be the hardest part, with influences coming from family, friends, and tradition. Maybe your mother-in-law is pushing hard for you to honor your great-aunt Mildred. DO NOT FEEL PRESSURE. I repeat, DO NOT FEEL PRESSURE! I have found that moms today are more obsessed with baby naming than ever before. Maybe it is because it is the one thing in your pregnancy that you can control. Well, almost. My husband and I immediately agreed on . . . absolutely nothing. It was clear we had completely opposite tastes in names. I pitched the names Aiden and Joel; he was holding out for Ace and Dino. He determined if he liked a name by testing how it would sound being announced at a pro ball game: "And now up . . . Ace Dat . . . !" I didn't have time to check into the latest baby-name trends; I was too busy convincing my husband that no matter how much he begged or bribed, we were not going to name our son Ace. Today the Internet has made it easier than ever to research (aka obsess) about your baby's name.

> "When picking a name, yell it three times really loud out the window and see if you still like it. No matter which name you choose, you will be saying it fifty to a hundred times a day, and most likely in a loud voice!"
>
> —My Mom

The Chinese believe that choosing the baby's name is extremely important. They feel one's name could influence everything that happens in one's life. (No pressure, huh?)

The Name Voyager (at www.babynamewizard.com) is the most popular place on the web to check the popularity of the name you love—for this week at least.

Today it seems we are being judged by our kids' names more often. Surprisingly popular names carry a bit of a stigma. A cool, hip baby name seems to be another status/style marker like having the latest Marc Jacobs bag . . . or hip pair of jeans. Growing up Jessica, I got used to my last name or initial always being tacked

> *"Always end the name of your child with a vowel, so that when you yell, the name will carry."*
> —Bill Cosby

on, because my best friend throughout high school was named Jessica too. My son introduces himself to people as Gabriel D. So far every year in school there has been more than one Gabriel in his class. You may like classic names. You may like annoyingly popular names. You may like outrageous names like Cabinet. Or you may be searching for the next amazing name no one has thought of. Whatever you like, remember it is your choice. Relax, it doesn't matter what anyone else thinks; you are the one who is going to be saying it . . . or screaming it, for the next twenty-plus years.

Keep It Simple

My husband and I were at our favorite Thai restaurant, which we frequented when we were dating, trying to come up with a name for our first son. My husband half-jokingly stated, "How about Ty?" I said, "I love it! That's it!"

—Sara Holliday,
fitness expert and mom to Ty and Kaden

During the baby-naming process, my husband and I must have batted around hundreds of names. It's amazing how names carry with them your associations with certain people. This one reminds you of that girl who was mean to you in third grade; another combined with your last name makes saying *rubber baby bumpers* easy. Or you finally come across a name you both like but find out it means "difficult child."

I've come up with a process to try that might help you avoid a number of naming pitfalls:

1. Write down all the names that have meant something to you or your spouse—and then cross out any that produce hives.

2. Check out the online baby-name sites for additional inspiration. You can check by nationality, meaning, or popularity.

3. Sit with mutually agreeable names for a few days . . . try them out, write them down, and secretly test them out on other babies.

4. If all else fails, walk through a bookstore, pick a book at random, open to any page, and choose the first name (gender appropriate) that you see. That's trusting to fate!

5. If you have other children, or nieces and nephews, for fun ask them what they think you should name the baby. You never know,

they may come up with a winner—although some names I've heard from siblings are Dora the Explorer, Rainbowhead, and Jelly Bean. My friend's son Rob suggested they name the new baby Rob the Second!

"Two hours after having my son, the phone in the hospital started ringing. Everyone had his or her own suggestions for a baby name. Not wanting to offend anyone, I chose one on my own."
—Victoria Pericon, *Savvy Mommy*

My husband and I were having trouble choosing a name. I was told "the baby whispers its name to you. If you listen carefully, the baby will tell you." Apparently that is exactly what happened! I was in New York for business and up late searching the Internet for names. I came across the name Wylder and loved it. I texted it to my husband and he texted right back "I love it." The very next day his mother called to tell us she thought she found a cute name we would like: "Wilder." That was it. He was telling us his name!
—Tricia Fisher,
owner Treehouse Social Club and
mom to Hudson, Holden, and Wylder

Decoy Names

When you are pregnant, everyone and their sister are going to suggest names to you. And then they are going to tell you how stupid and wrong the name you most love is. So instead of telling them the real name, I always liked to have a list of decoys available. Depending on the people, I made the list more or less believable. For friends, I just went with some of the most popular names out there, the Ethans and Rileys. It shut them up pretty fast. For the in-laws, I went with more far-out name choices like Cosmo and Desdemona. It toughened them up for the less conventional names we were likely to actually choose. After the baby is born, few people will actually have the nerve to comment on the name in a negative fashion. And if they do, then you can think of a new name to call them.

—Ciaran Blumenfeld,
writer and Hot Moms Club member

Beyond Jennifer & Jason, Madison & Montana and *Cool Names for Babies* by Pamela Redmond Satran and Linda Rosenknantz are two of the hottest books you can use to begin your name search. Their site, www.babynamebible.com, has a feature called the Alternator, where you can plug in names you love but are afraid are overused. The site then provides you with names you might like instead that are similar, but different!

Bruce Lansky is the "Baby Name Guru." He writes reviews of celebrity baby names for the Hot Moms Club site, and his baby-naming advice and commentary have been published in thousands of newspapers, magazines, and websites. He makes great points in his book *5 Star Baby Name Advisor*, where he not only lists names but also gives you their pros and cons. He brings up great points and things you might never have thought of regarding the names you are thinking about.

> We decided to name our second daughter Phoebe and told our families on Christmas Day. After a whole day of hearing everyone refer to our unborn child by this name, we just weren't feeling it anymore—it was like we took the name on a test drive.
> —Tara Sebastiano,
> mom of Casey and Ellie and
> Hot Moms Club member

The Internet has made it easier than ever to research, focus, and fixate about the name you give your child. Ultimately, it's your choice. The name of your baby is the decision of you and your partner, guided by your personal beliefs. Period. You will be saying this name for the rest of your life, so make sure it is a sound you like and that it gives a bit of meaning to your child's life, either through a family association or through the name's actual meaning. We ended up naming our son Gabriel, and he is truly our little "angel" . . . well, most of the time!

JOURNAL—MONTH FIVE

1. You know you're still you in mind, body, and spirit, even though your body is doing a change-up. Think of your fashion MO and how can you maintain your joy for color and style even with the bump.

_____

_____

_____

_____

_____

_____

_____

_____

_____

_____

_____

_____

_____

_____

2. Take a picture of yourself in your best preg fashion and paste it here.

_____

_____

_____

_____

_____

_____

_____

_____

_____

_____

_____

_____

_____

_____

_____

_____

_____

_____

3. Hey, what was that? Record the first kicks of your baby—where, when, how hard?

_____

_____

_____

_____

_____

_____

_____

_____

_____

_____

_____

_____

_____

_____

_____

_____

_____

_____

_____

_____

_____

4. What baby names do you like today?

_____

_____

_____

_____

_____

_____

_____

_____

_____

_____

_____

_____

_____

_____

_____

_____

_____

_____

_____

_____

_____

5. What suggested baby named have you heard?

_____
_____
_____
_____
_____
_____
_____
_____
_____
_____
_____
_____
_____
_____
_____
_____
_____
_____
_____
_____
_____

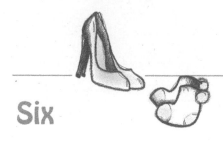

Six

Get Glowing

Imagine staying up all night, then running a marathon,
then doing three hundred loads of laundry
and raking leaves off a football field all in one day.
How tired would you be? That's how tired
I felt every day in my first trimester.

—Jenny McCarthy from her book, *Belly Laughs*

Yes, for most women this is the point during pregnancy when you start to ache a little more, move a little slower, and feel a whole lot fatter. Your body is adjusting to weight, water, and hormones, and—though sometimes you feel absolutely fabulous—other times you'll find yourself a little stuffed and uncomfortable, like a Thanksgiving turkey.

It's time to lift your spirits, glow and beam, and treat yourself right! Think of this time as an opportunity to take a tour of your senses, with special attention to taste, smell, and touch. Also, give yourself a chance to experience your body in gentle ways that keep you breathing, stretching, and moving.

Mama-Massage

Recruit that man into a massage! I know that a simple ten-minute foot massage gave me all the relief in the world when I was pregnant—and if I got the full shoulder treatment, I was in heaven. But as we know, not all men were created equal in the massage department. If your partner doesn't have "magic hands," investigate the pregnancy massage specialists in your area. Not only will you feel better but the benefits can also include reduced joint pain, better digestion, and improved circulation—all things that help you and your baby. Prenatal massage packages are available at most major spas today. If ever there was a time to treat yourself to a day of pampering, this is it!

Pamper Yourself at Home

If a day at the spa is out of your budget, or if you just prefer to relax in your home, you can still give yourself the royal treatment. There are so many ways to pamper yourself at home during pregnancy—and don't forget to encourage some pampering from others. The words *massage, gourmet,* and *sensuous* come to mind—and don't think that you don't deserve it or that you'll wait until you have your old body back. No way! There are many ways to relax and unwind without even leaving your house.

First things first—get yourself a "spa uniform." In order to truly feel pampered and glowing, you must be comfortable. I don't mean to get all Hugh Hefner on you, but invest in a cozy robe—one that is soft and feels fabulous on, one that you never want to take off. While you are at it, find yourself a pair of snuggly slippers. You can't feel serene if you're not comfortable.

The Little Giraffe (www.littlegiraffe.com) and Barefoot Dreams have the most scrumptious robes (www.barefootdreams.com). Also check out KooKoo Bear Kids (www.kookoobearkids.com) for the softest poly chenille robe selection.

Golf Ball Foot Massage

"Hit Nausea with a hole in one." What you will need is a bowl big enough for your feet to fit side by side, two towels, two golf balls, and mandarin or tangerine essential oils. Put six drops of the essential oil in the bowl and fill it with warm water. Put the bowl on the floor in front of a comfy chair with a towel on either side and a golf ball on each towel. Soak your feet for a few minutes and then take your left foot out and roll the golf ball over the towel using the arch of your foot, then switch feet. Add more warm water as it cools.

This treatment starts off with a wonderfully fragrant foot soak containing mandarin essential oil, which is known to relieve all kinds of stomach upsets including morning sickness. And rolling your feet over golf balls will pep up even the most tired of toes.

—from *Spa Mama*, by Stacey Denney

If this is not your first pregnancy and you have little ones running around, you may find it a lot more challenging to soak your feet for a few minutes. We all know kids need to have their fingers and toenails clipped, so incorporate a little spa time for all into this task. Set out warm bowls of sudsy water for you and the kids. Have everyone soak her or his feet for a few minutes, and then it's time to trim. It's all in how you "train" them. My advice: start young. My son was so used to this routine that when my mother went to cut his nails, he said, "Wait, we have to soak them first!" Whether this is your first child or your tenth, as a mom even just a few minutes of peace can leave you feeling victorious and ready for anything the day throws your way.

Turn Your Bathroom into a Mini-Oasis

Bath time is not just for kids. One of the most pampering pleasures in life is soaking in a luxurious bath with pleasing scents. Baths increase body circulation and relax muscles. Soaking yourself in water cleanses more than just your body; it also unwinds and rejuvenates your spirit and soul. Your muscles loosen up in its warmth as the water works its calming miracles. It is easier than you think to create a gourmet bath experience. Add scented candles to create a peaceful mood and aura, day or night. Play your favorite soft music. Place a few drops of your favorite scented essential oils into the tub. Lavender before bed will help you sleep. Coconut oil helps lift your mood. Use citrus for when you're feeling ill. Try Epsom salts if your back is aching.

A Little Bubbly

Bubble baths visually remind people of their childhood or make them feel frivolous and spoiled. Dropping flower petals or flower tops can also make the bath seem extra special. To appeal to all of your senses, add a few drops of food coloring into the bath, as colors can affect your mood. Blues and greens create a sense of tranquility. Pink also relaxes you. Purple will make you feel comforted and creative. Yellow recharges and energizes you. Red and orange arouse passion and excitement.

If you have little ones, carve out time to take a luscious bath when they are in bed. Enlist the help of your hubby or hire a sitter to take the kids out so you can steal some rest and relaxation time. YOU DESERVE IT!—and your family deserves to have you at your best.

Mama Scent-sibility

Increased sensitivity to the world around you seems to be a by-product of pregnancy. Maybe it's the body's way of reminding us to take care of ourselves . . . or maybe it's nature's way of reminding us what it's like to be a newborn! Babies are extraordinarily sensitive too. In any case, the Hot Moms Club has a few suggestions for keeping yourself happily sensitive, sensible, and sen-sotic! For example, use great-smelling shampoos, creams and body washes, candles, or fresh flowers. Aromas subtly influence your behavior; mood and energy levels can make time and work go so much easier. During pregnancy, our brains are sensitive— really sensitive—to smells. It's those hormones again; even the slightest whiff of broccoli or A1 steak sauce can send you running from the room. So treat yourself to pleasant scents.

BUMP ON A BUDGET

You don't have to spend a fortune to smell and feel great. Suave's Exhale line of lotions and body washes (www.suave.com) are affordable and come in a variety of great-smelling scents, including lavender vanilla, cinnamon, sandalwood (my favorite), and lime verbosa.

ECO-MINDED MAMA

Created by Epicuren and in association with Anne Geddes, Epicuren Baby skin care line for babies is the first to help in development and immune functions. Infused with Episencial aromatherapy oil blends to promote bonding and awakening of the senses (www.episencial.com).

Get Therapy—Aromatherapy

Check out your local health food store for natural and organic essential oils. There are plenty of relaxing blends; use the testers and find your favorites. Essential oils are not the same as perfumes or artificially created fragrances; they come from real plants and are the most potent and concentrated extracts of various parts of flowers, fruits, leaves, spices, roots, and woods. They have therapeutic psychological and physical benefits. Mint, lavender, and chamomile seem to be popular with pregnant women since they have calming effects, but your favorites could be very different. I couldn't stand the smell of roses during pregnancy, but I loved the scent of pineapple. It's all very individual. Once you find a scent you like, add a few drops of the oil into your garbage can, drain, or vacuum bag filter—or use a diffuser to keep a room in a blissful state. Remember, though: some essential oils are powerful, so they should be diluted with water and never directly applied to the skin or swallowed. Make sure to follow all of the directions, and if you are unsure, talk to your doctor.

Wax On, Wax Off

At this time, your belly may be feeling a bit itchy. Keep it lubricated with lotion by rubbing it on in a circular motion. Sensuous healing crèmes with help make you feel a little more "comfortable in your own skin." Since you will be reapplying several times a day, warming the lotion will make it a pleasant and soothing experience. Also, because your skin is expanding and stretching so rapidly, stretch marks are likely to occur. (Don't shoot the messenger!) Rub cocoa butter and vitamin E oil on every day.

Tummy Honey, found at www.mothersintuition.com, is a popular choice for keeping your belly moisturized while minimizing and helping to prevent stretch marks. Using a soft loofah to scrub off and exfoliate dead skin reveals more vibrant and soft skin and regenerates new cells, thereby lessening the appearance or chances of marks. There are a lot of products out there that claim to prevent stretch marks or cure them completely, but don't get too excited—there is no miracle cure yet. The majority—75 to 90 percent—of pregnant moms end up with some sort of marks. Stretch marks occur because the skin is stretched to the limits of its elasticity; you may be lucky and escape, or you may find them on your belly, butt, or breasts. Just be prepared: even if you religiously apply creams and lotions, you may still end up with a few. I did. The good news is that they fade over time and they appear in places that can be easily hidden with clothes. You, your belly, and your whole body will feel smoother and less irritated if you continually moisturize and exfoliate. It can be a fun and sensuous experience to have your man rub lotions on your belly the next time you are feeling a *bit-itchy*!

There are plenty of products out there to help you feel pampered and more confident about your changing shape. Mama Mio (www.mamamio.com) is a Hot

"Think of stretch marks as pregnancy service stripes."

—Joyce Armor

Moms Club favorite. They have kits and creams for every stage of your pregnancy, and every inch of your growing body. They have a selection of all-natural stretch mark oil, butter, serum, and cream. Their popular kits, Bootcamp for your Boobs and Bootcamp for your Butt, have all you need to help firm those expanding areas.

ECO-MINDED MAMA

It is believed that everything you apply to your skin ends up in your bloodstream and passed on to your developing baby. It is more important than ever to be conscious of the products you use on your face and tummy during your pregnancy. The more natural and eco-friendly, the better.

Belli (www.belliskincare.com) uses organic ingredients and is free of parabens, preservatives, and synthetic fragrances.

Mambino Organics (www.mambinoorganics.com) has a great 9 Month Journey pack and a Bun in the Oven skin care package affordable for $44. Mambino has real ingredients harvested organically from botanicals around the world.

I just love Earth Mama Angel Baby (www.earth mamaangelbaby.com). This company has organic products for any need you might have, from pregnancy to delivery and postpartum. The Mother of all Pregnancy Gift Baskets has everything you will need.

Veda Mama (www.vedamama.com) luxury line of natural skin care starts at $75 for a three-ounce bottle.

Bébéologie (at www.maternitique.com) is a completely natural baby skin care line for mom and is gentle enough to use on infants. Complete product set is $250.

Bringing Sexy Back—To Your Belly

For as long as women have been having babies, moms around the globe have searched for the fastest techniques (fad diets and pricey exercise regimes aside) to get their pre-preggo bods back. I wish someone had told me about wrapping my tummy post-pregnancy. In many cultures around the world, belly binding is considered a normal way to tone up. After my son was born, my stomach looked like a flab of elephant skin. It went away eventually and I got my figure back, but products like The Belly Bandit (www.bellybandit.com), specially made wraps to tighten your tummy, help hold everything in place. Many of our moms rave about them and the results. Several also said it reduced the pressure on their backs and made the healing process much easier after a C-section. Whether for comfort or vanity, or a little of both, this product is worth trying and sharing with all your friends.

Although belly wrapping has been practiced in the East for centuries, Western women and Hollywood celebrities are only now jumping on board with the process. Actress, model, and *Dancing with the Stars*

Get Glowing   201

champion Brooke Burke credits her rockin' post-baby bikini bod (after four children) to the ancient tradition of post-pregnancy belly wrapping. She was so excited to share her secret with other women that she created her own product, Tauts Belly Wrap, which she sells on her site, www.babooshbaby.com.

*Please note: Tauts and Belly Bandits should NEVER be worn during pregnancy. These are for getting your belly back in shape *after* your kids are born.

ECO-MINDED MAMA
Belly Bandit also offers an all-natural bamboo selection of belly wraps.

BUMP ON A BUDGET
How You Feeling—Hot, Hot, Hot?

If it is midsummer and you can't escape the heat, your two-dollar solution is a spritz bottle. Pick one up at your local drugstore, fill it with water, and add a few pinches of lemon or lime juice (or you can put a few drops of your favorite scented oil in there as well). Keep it at arm's length and spray. Cover yourself with the cool, refreshing mist. This simple thing will help you feel really recharged. If you have little ones, give them the task of spritzing and cooling your arms, legs, and belly. They'll have fun, and you'll feel refreshed, at least for a little while!

One of the Most Magnificent Words: Naptime

You don't have to wait until your child is born to enjoy naptime. Rest to relax, nap to revive, and sleep to rejuvenate: all three are important components to make it through these last months. Resting is that five-to-fifteen-minute break of literally putting up your feet. Perhaps you can catch up on your favorite magazines or listen to music, but whatever choice you make, let yourself relax into a comfortable chair and refuse to run for anything . . . not even the phone.

I recall having waves of tiredness hit me about this time. Not ordinary tired, but that dead-on-your-feet tired, when I finally understood "too tired to lift a finger." I definitely needed a bit more than just a little rest, but *nap* was still a foreign word to me. Before pregnancy, I was not the type to even consider sleeping during the day, but once I allowed myself the fifteen-to-thirty-minute snooze, I had so much more energy. So allow yourself the luxury of taking a nap every day. Sometimes this takes some self-convincing, because we're women and no matter how tired we are, we will always think of at least a dozen things that we could be doing instead. If you have other children, nap when they do.

And lastly, try to sleep your full eight hours. Sleep is the best way to rejuvenate your mind and body. Just keep in mind the effort your body is making to create a safe and healthy environment for your child—and know that your rest and reduced stress translate into a better beginning for your little one. Hint: sleep now, because you won't sleep once the baby comes!

All hail Yogi Poof (www.yogipoof.com)! These body pillows are a Hot Mom must-have. BabyAge.com (www.babyage.com) also has an affordable selection and variety of comfy body pillows to help make sleeping easier.

SOS: "Sleep on Side"

It is recommended to sleep on your left side. Sleeping on your left increases the amount of blood and nutrients that reach the placenta and your baby. If possible, avoid sleeping on your back, among other things it can cause backaches, hemorrhoids, can decrease circulation to your heart and baby, as your abdomen is resting on your intestines and major blood vessels.

BUMP ON A BUDGET

Hot Moms Club also loves the Luna Lullaby Bosom Baby (www.lunalullaby.com) It's a V-shaped pillow that lends great support for your tummy when you are lying down and is the perfect fit after the baby is born to use as a nursing and feeding pillow. They come in fashionable styles and colors too!

Kick up Your Feet!

Whether you are watching television, reading, or just chatting with family or friends, prop a pillow under your feet and put them up! This not only feels relaxing but also helps to prevent varicose or spider veins. Spanx (www.spanx.com) has a maternity line of support hose and thigh shapers. The nylon yarn stretches as your belly grows and provides support to your lower back and legs.

Move-ease

With a newborn, getting to the movies will be a bit of a challenge. Pregnancy is an ideal time to catch up on sleep AND those movies you have been meaning to see. Now, if your bladder rebels against sitting in a theater for two-plus hours, then a subscription to Netflix or Blockbuster at home may be the perfect solution. Really, is there anything cozier than curling up on your bed or couch with a fun movie? Get comfortable and treat yourself to a few buckets of popcorn and a new movie—or an old favorite. (Comedies are best to keep you in a relaxed, happy mood.)

Hot Moms Club's favorite pregnancy flicks:

1. *Nine Months*

2. *Baby Boom*

3. *She's Having a Baby*

4. *Due Date*

5. *Fools Rush In*

6. *Look Who's Talking*

7. *Knocked Up*

8. *Juno*

9. *Baby Mama*

10. *Waitress*

11. *Away We Go*

Amazon (www.amazon.com) even has a list of "Movies for Pregnancy Hormones," including a special edition of *Steel Magnolias* and *Beaches*. On the web, you can find *In the Motherhood* webisodes starring Leah Remini and Chelsea Handler (www.inthemotherhood.com). Anita Renfroe's *Total Momsense* has all of the classic mom-isms sung to the *William Tell* Overture and is one of the most popular downloads on YouTube. Watch for yourself.

Babes on TV: Some fun shows to watch to get you excited about your little one on the way:

> **On Discovery Health**—*Babies: Special Delivery; Birth Day; Deliver Me; Bringing Home Baby; Runway Moms*
> **TLC**—*A Baby Story*
> **We**—*Platinum Babies*

Pamper Yourself with a Book

About now you have probably read every pregnancy book and magazine on the shelves. Take time out to read a good book or a magazine that does not revolve around motherhood. You will not have the time to get lost in a good book for a long while after the baby is born, so carve out a few hours and grab an uplifting read. There is something refreshing about connecting to your imagination and to worlds outside your own—it brings joy, refreshment, confidence, and a sense of self that makes you feel hot because you're the smart, sexy woman you've always been.

A Little Grooming Goes a Long Way

It's no secret that when we look good, we feel good. Often during pregnancy we are so busy making sure we are eating healthy, getting to our doctor appointments on time, buying everything baby, and preparing for the new arrival that we forget to keep up with our beauty routines. There is something about having my nails done that makes me feel so beautiful and pampered. As you may be experiencing, it is getting more and more difficult to see your toes, let alone paint them. If

"I know this is going to sound corny, but I first became happy with the way I look when I became a mother."
—Angelina Jolie

this is something that usually makes you feel good, see if your man will paint them for you, or treat yourself to a pedicure. In fact, schedule a full beauty day, complete with a haircut, wax, nails, the works—anything that will make you feel pulled together. And forget about feeling guilty—remember, you (and by extension, your little one) deserve a completely stress-free day!

A final note: remember to make sure that the salon you visit is well ventilated. Breathing in fumes is not good for you or your baby. All-natural salons and hair coloring are safe alternatives to chemical hair dyes with ammonia, which should be avoided during your pregnancy. One of Hollywood's hottest hairstylists, Susan Henry, developed a hair color line that is all natural and ammonia free. Check it out at www.susanhenry-ncp.com.

The Russians have many traditions. One is that they feel visibly pregnant women shouldn't cut their hair.

En-lighten?

A healthy, bright smile can make you look years younger, and teeth whitening has grown intensely in popularity. If this is something you do once or twice a year, you may be questioning whether it is safe or not for your baby. As always, ask your doctor and consult your dentist. Although there are no studies to link to any problems, none of the dentists I spoke to would perform teeth bleaching procedures on pregnant women, citing unnecessary liability. They did, however, recommend teeth cleanings to remove stains, whitening toothpastes, and using baking soda as an alternative whitening solution. So, until more research is done, it's better safe than sorry!

Face It!

Some women say that their skin never looked better than when they were pregnant. Others, prone to the surging hormonal activity of pregnancy, say the opposite. I escaped morning sickness but not the breakouts—my skin really took the pregnancy hard. Consult a dermatologist and find a cleansing routine and mask that will help eliminate any acne, while also helping your skin glow and feel revitalized. Mud masks are a lot of fun. My husband used to make fun of me when I wore one until I convinced him to try it. He was surprised how much he loved the way it made his face feel afterward, and it became a fun weekly ritual. Also, if you have little ones at home, a great way to combine play and your beauty routine is to put on your "monster" mask (as my son would call it) and run around the house chasing the kids. Talk about multitasking!

Cha Cha Cha Changes . . .

Aside from acne, changes in your hormone levels can also create changes in the pigment of your skin. You may be experiencing a darkening of your freckles, moles, and facial skin in general—also known as "the mask of pregnancy." Your sexual organs will most likely enlarge and darken, including your nipples and labia (lips of your vagina). And, of course, you may be noticing that dark line in the center of your belly as well. Don't be alarmed. While all of these things may be unavoidable during pregnancy, they often all go away or fade after birth. You also might be seeing strange little pieces or flaps of skin appearing under your armpits or on your neck. These skin tags—while they may be unattractive—are quite normal and harmless and can be removed by your doctor after birth.

Using sunblock is always a beauty must, but during pregnancy your skin is ultrasensitive, and using a strong sunscreen is especially important, as the sun can cause brown spots and increase the chance of getting the "mask of pregnancy."

Things aren't all bad, though; some women find their prenatal complexion to be absolutely radiant. Your hair and nails are said to grow faster and stronger, and, because blood flow is increased during pregnancy (including the tiny vessels just below the skin's surface), your face and body should have a warm, rosy glow.

A quick beauty pick-me-up: To enhance your natural pregnancy glow, brush on a little shimmer powder to your cheekbones, chest, neckline, arms, and legs. Use lip balm and gloss with a high shine.

Life of the Potty

Tired of the prescriptive eating and drinking "for two" with not a lot of fun or frills? Well, who says you can't change the pace and serve up some tasty (nonalcoholic) cocktails and delicious canapés at a Hot-Mom-to-be soiree? You don't have to wait until the baby shower to get some friends together. Hold a "Homemade Happy Hour." Granted, your party may include mostly women from your Lamaze set—a wild bunch packing babies and hemorrhoids—but you can still wow them with the taste of these yummy "mock"-tails.

HOT MOM MARTINI

✿ 2 ounces fresh pomegranate juice

✿ 1 ounce of lemonade

✿ Splash of pineapple juice

✿ Splash of Sprite or 7-Up

✿ Combine and serve in a martini glass with sugar rim.

MOJITO MAMA

✿ 2 ounces bottled Mojito mix (presweetened)

✿ 1 ounce sweet and sour mix or lemonade

✿ Splash of Sprite or 7-Up

✿ Splash of soda water

✿ Serve in a tall glass on ice with sugar rim. Garnish with lime. (You can also add fresh crushed mint leaves in the bottom of glass if you'd like.)

I DREAM OF PIÑA COLADAS

The piña colada nutritional drink from Angel Milk (www.theangelmilkgroup.com) is absolute genius. It tastes like a piña colada, but it's actually good for you and your baby, with high protein, soothing herbs, and all the right vitamins. What's great about something like Angel Milk is that it's in powdered form—so you can take it with you wherever you go. And if the Lamaze Moms want to add piña coladas to the cocktail list, just whip up a batch, pour it on ice, add a pineapple slice— and you are ready to go.

PREGGATINIS ANYONE?

Preggatinis: Mixology for the Mom-To-Be, by Natalie Bovis-Nelson, features more than seventy-five original recipes designed with the fun-loving preggie party girl in mind. Natalie, a Hot Moms Club contributor, has mixed signature cocktails for celebrity-studded events; she agreed to spill one of her scrumptious concoctions from her book with us.

WHITE HOT MAMA

Most men find the mother of their unborn child hotter than before. Snuggle up and revel in the beauty of your yin and yang with this hot, creamy glass of decadence —with a kick!

- ❂ 1/2 teaspoon ground dried ancho chili powder

- ❂ 1/2 teaspoon vanilla extract (optional)

- ❂ 2 tablespoons white hot chocolate cocoa powder

- ❂ 1 teaspoon honey

- ❂ 1 cup whole milk

- ❂ 2 tablespoons caramel sauce

Drizzle caramel sauce around the inside of a heat-resistant mug, particularly around the inside of the rim. Mix the remaining ingredients in a small saucepan and bring to a vigorous simmer, over medium heat. Then, reduce the heat and continue to simmer for five minutes, stirring constantly. Let the mixture cool to slightly above room temperature and gently pour into the heat-resistant glass or mug. Yum!

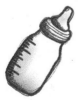

Wine, Yes. Whine, Oh No!

Through our Hot Moms Club website, we've found an all-natural sparkling drink called Vignette Wine Country Soda, which is made from premium wine grapes. For you moms who crave the taste of a nice glass of wine, you can now get your drink on anytime during the day or night. These special sodas come in glass bottles with twist-off tops and are available in Pinot Noir, Chardonnay, and Rosé. They're 100 percent alcohol free, and you can find them at www.winecountrysoda.com. Trader Joe's also carries a sparkling pomegranate juice that makes a yummy and healthy champagne substitute.

Like a Virgin

Let's face it, if you're really craving your favorite cocktail, make it a virgin and pretend!

Sweeeeeeet!

Chocolate is one of the most commonly craved foods of pregnant women. If you are a chocoholic, then you will be very excited to know that there are many benefits to indulging your craving. Several studies reveal that eating chocolate during pregnancy is good for you and may even produce a happier baby. Chocolate is rich in flavonoids, which are plant compounds with potent antioxidant properties that enhance our cardiovascular and immune systems.

Switch to the "Dark Side"

The way cocoa beans are grown and processed determines how much of the original flavonoid content is retained. Milk chocolates loaded with sugar, additives, and fillers are not good for you or your little one. Dark and bitter chocolate has twice as many flavonoids as sweet milk chocolate. Unsweetened cocoa powder starts out twice as high in flavonoids as dark chocolate, but when it's diluted with milk or water and sugar, the flavonoid total decreases to half of that in milk chocolate. Studies also found that drinking milk at the same time as chocolate cancels out its health benefits.

Health by Chocolate (www.healthbychocolate.com) and the Protein Bakery (www.theproteinbakery.com) are great places to order indulgent yummy chocolate treats that are actually good for you!

Power Snacks

What we put inside ourselves affects how we feel on the outside, and more and more studies are concluding that the nutritional value in the food we eat affects our growing fetus. So treat yourself to some delicious treats or "power snacks." When I was pregnant, I had trail mix with me at all times. Mix a bag of your favorite nuts, seeds, dried fruit, and some dark chocolate chips, and munch throughout the day to stay balanced and energized . . . go nuts!

Eda-mommy!

Edamame is a green vegetable also known as soybeans. You can eat them alone as a fun snack. Just heat them up in the microwave and add a pinch of salt, or eat them cold with a spritz of lemon juice. Add them to salad, pasta, or stir-fry for an extra shot of protein.

Fun Fruits

Fruit always seems to taste better when it is either frozen or dipped in a delicious sauce. Frozen red grapes or banana slices make a refreshing and healthy snack. Sliced apples dipped in natural peanut butter (avoid peanut butter with additives and sugar—the only ingredients should be nuts!) and strawberries dipped in yogurt or cottage cheese drizzled with honey are yummy too. All of these healthy treats satisfy your sweet tooth while giving your baby the nutrition he or she needs. Fruit to go!

Crispy Green has freeze-dried fruit in packets, which make light crispy snacks—perfect for the working mom-to-be or mom on the go (www.crispygreen.com).

Feeling Crappy?

It's hard to feel comfortable and relaxed when you are all blocked up. Constipation is common during pregnancy because of the iron in your prenatal vitamins, the increase in the hormone progesterone (which slows the movement of food through the digestive system), and, as the baby grows, your uterus expanding—putting pressure on your rectum and intestines. Not the most enticing visual, but facts are facts, and you can't feel Zen when you are feeling *crappy*! You can prevent and treat constipation by drinking lots of water; engaging in simple exercise like a daily walk; and increasing your fiber intake by eating more bran, fruits, whole grain breads, beans, etc. If you are still uncomfortable, ask your doctor about over-the-counter stool softeners and switching you to a supplement with a lower iron content.

Waddle You Know

Waddle ya know . . . yep. It's a little difficult doing your normal exercise routine with a bowling ball between your legs. Some women continue aerobics right up till delivery, but most make some adjustments to their exercise routine.

Before I became pregnant, I was very physically active. I was an athlete all through school and loved to run, and I figured I'd keep up the routine right through pregnancy. I know, I know, running is not the most popular recommendation for pregnant women . . . just keep reading. The doctor gave me the thumbs-up to continue running, but I have to admit that after the first ultrasound, when I saw how the baby tossed and turned like a fish in a bag when I merely laughed, I could only imagine how jostled he would be if I ran. So I took up the wild sport of walking.

> "When I was pregnant my doctor told me to exercise a little less than I normally would. Uh, that would be a coma."
> —Stephanie Blum, comedian, mom of three, and Hot Moms Club member

I mapped my course (two laps around my block), and, armed with my Walkman (yikes—today an iPod!), a stopwatch, and a bottle of water, I took off on my daily hike. I timed my revolutions like I was in the Olympics, keeping track of my time and keeping my heart rate at a reasonable low-aerobic level.

The stopwatch may seem a bit over the top, but trust me, it's the fun part. In the beginning it won't be a big deal, but by the end of your pregnancy it will be downright hilarious when it takes you fourteen minutes to waddle past your neighbor's house. Okay, I'm exaggerating, but in my final days I swear I was lapped by an eighty-year-old in a walker.

Kicking Butt vs. Kicking Back

The thing is this: I recommend that you—as a mom-to-be, no matter what your athletic background—find some physical release that works for you. Walking is great because it keeps you fit during your pregnancy and helps your mood. For me, it was so relaxing, listening to my music and just taking in the neighborhood. This was the most peaceful time of the day, when I could really think. And my doctor said that walking until the end of my term helped get the baby in position and helped me dilate easier.

Exercise is essential for promoting the health and well-being of pregnant women and their babies. Not only will exercise during pregnancy increase stamina but it will also reduce the risk of excess weight gain during the months leading up to delivery. It will also promote rapid post-pregnancy weight loss. If you are currently doing Pilates, just let your instructor know you are pregnant. If you are strength training, you may continue, just lessen the weight as the pregnancy progresses. If you are a cardio junkie, double-check with your doctor on where to keep your heart rate. Even if you never exercised before, get moving! This is no time to sit on your bottom and watch it spread.

I'm not saying that it's time to get in the

best shape of your life. But I will say you will feel more alive and energized. Exercise helps to relax both the mind and the body by releasing adrenaline and other hormones, which improve sleeping patterns and mood. Because pregnancy is a highly complex physiological state, women must first consult with their physicians before beginning any fitness program. Being guided by personal trainers who specialize in working with the pregnant population is also beneficial. Trainers are equipped with the knowledge and experience to develop a routine specialized to your personal needs.

—Anita Pressman,
professional fitness trainer
for over ten years and mother of Devin

HOT MOMS CLUB'S FAVORITE PRENATAL WORKOUT VIDEOS TO KEEP YOU FIT AND MOTIVATED

Gabrielle Reese: Fit and Healthy Prenatal Workout (www.gotogabby.com)
Anna Getty's Pre & Post Natal Yoga Workout (www.annagetty.com)
Tracey Mallett's *3-in-1 Patented Pregnancy System*, which combines Pilates, yoga, and strength training (www.traceymallett.com)

Jennifer Nicole Lee's Fabulously Fit Moms workout DVD series (www.fabulouslyfitmoms.com)

Sara Holliday's Fit for Mom collection (www.fitbysara.com)

Belly Dance: Prenatal Fitness and Dance Instruction Program with Naia

Take a Load Off

Swimming is another ideal sport for Hot Moms. If this appeals to you but you don't have a pool, make fast friends with someone who does or find a membership pool near you where you can do nice long laps. The water relieves any heaviness or pressure from extra weight, the repetition is relaxing, and if you have a tendency to get warm during exercise, the cool water makes you feel as if you're barely breaking a sweat.

If you already have a fitness club membership, check the list to see if there are any pregnancy classes. If not, you probably can't continue the heavy-duty cardio-kickboxing-weights-and-hula workout, but there are milder classes that can still keep you fit.

For city moms whose chance of taking a relaxing walk down the block or a private swim are as realistic as finding a *Kiss Me, I'm Irish* sweatshirt in Madonna's closet, I suggest yoga. Prenatal yoga is the perfect way to stay fit and relaxed: not only do you gently move and stretch all those aching places but yoga also encourages awareness of muscles and movement that will translate to all areas of life. This can really help a year down the line, when baby lifting becomes your favorite sport. Furthermore, depending on the teacher or type of practice, yoga can also teach focus and relaxation techniques, along with our next subject, breathing.

Learning to BREATHE

Ready. Blow out the air. All of it. Then let those ribs expand, really expand, and take air in. Yes! That's it, you're breathing. Funny, isn't it—that we would actually have to learn to breathe? Something that seems so obvious, something that we do every second, something we take completely for granted—and yet learning to be more conscious of the process of breathing can be a powerful force in relaxation and alertness. Also, breath awareness is an enormously helpful tool in labor! Your delivery classes will undoubtedly teach some breathing routines—and yoga teachers will guide you through deep breathing techniques—but if you're not getting that assistance, just try the following:

First, just breathe normally and observe what happens. Is your belly rising and falling, or is the rise and fall in your upper chest only? Is anything restricting your breathing—clothing, posture, emotions? Is your breathing regular and steady at a rate of about ten to sixteen times per minute?

Next, get in a comfortable position, either lying down or standing, or sitting in a chair with back straight but relaxed. Observe your breathing for a few moments. Has it changed?

Next, consciously control your breathing. Take a slow, deep breath, expanding your lungs fully. Watch your navel area rise upward (or outward if you are sitting or standing) as far as it can possibly go. Exhale slowly and imagine your navel area sinking toward your backbone. Empty out your lungs completely. Relax and begin to draw in the next breath. Do this slowly several times. Don't do this too fast or you will hyperventilate. How does this feel compared to your previous observations?

Simple breathing practices like these will keep you calm, reduce distractions, and give you tools for becoming the BMP, the Best Mom Possible—not perfect, but at least aware of when you are breathing and in your body.

On to the Last Trimester

Too often in everyday life we're in our heads, thinking about that never-ending to-do list and figuring out the next set of problems. Let this time during your pregnancy reintroduce you to your senses and to enjoying your body. This is something you can continue to practice throughout your life and share with your children and loved ones.

1. What are your three least favorite, body-jerking smells right now? What are the three soothing scents that chill you out?

_____

_____

_____

_____

_____

_____

_____

_____

_____

_____

_____

_____

_____

_____

_____

_____

_____

_____

_____

_____

_____

2. Describe exactly what is necessary to get your partner to give you that all-important foot massage.

_____

_____

_____

_____

_____

_____

_____

_____

_____

_____

_____

_____

_____

_____

_____

_____

_____

_____

_____

_____

_____

3. Make plans for a low-stress gathering of friends (pregnant or not) where the drinks and food are tantalizing, and the mood is cool!

_____

_____

_____

_____

_____

_____

_____

_____

_____

_____

_____

_____

_____

_____

_____

_____

4. What things make you feel pampered and beautiful? Make sure you find time to do those things thio month.

_____

_____

_____

_____

_____

_____

_____

_____

_____

_____

_____

_____

_____

_____

_____

_____

_____

_____

5. We all know that exercise and diet plans don't always go as planned. Engage your sense of humor and describe your successes AND your less-than-stellar moments.

_____

_____

_____

_____

_____

_____

_____

_____

_____

_____

_____

_____

_____

_____

_____

_____

_____

_____

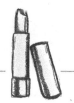

Seven

Keeping It Hot
When You're About to Pop!

I can't stand those people who love to issue ridiculous warnings before you have kids; you know the ones. They feel the need to let you know how tough having kids is on your marriage—with the whole loss of freedom, no alone time . . . blah-blah. How about fewer downers and a few more "You are the hottest seven-months-pregnant woman I've ever seen!"

—Stefanie Wilder-Taylor,

author of *Sippy Cups Are Not for Chardonnay*

and *Naptime Is the New Happy Hour*

Okay, when you are seven months pregnant, making love can look more like a hilarious circus act than an erotic one. Every couple is different; the key is to find and make a connection that's fun and enjoyable for you both. It may take some time, and it may adjust with your mood—one minute you feel like a sexy bombshell (or "mom"-shell) and then the next you may be overwhelmed by the many changes in your body and concerns about intercourse impacting the baby. Or maybe you believe your man isn't interested. Or maybe you're tired and uncomfortable, and your libido has moved to the next state. Trust me, there are ways to deal with all of this! The Hot Moms Club was established to prove that being a mom and being sexy aren't mutually exclusive, that you and your family benefit from a mother who not only provides care and comfort but who is also witty, funny, sensual, and confident in her body. Even now, especially now, with "the bump."

But if you've stalled out and can't seem to get back to the fantasizing and fun, remember there are two parts to the equation: one is convincing yourself that you still are a sexy goddess and the other is reminding your man that there's room for spice with this new you. There's magic in coming together once you both remember how good your bodies can feel. And there's a good chance that when you do light the flame, your increased sensitivity will ignite with better (or more) orgasms. Who knew?

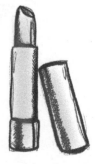

Sex and the Pregnant Woman

Okay, ladies, so here's the scoop on how a bun-in-the-oven just might interruptus your coitus—or not—depending on your body. The thing is this: hormone changes during pregnancy can impact libido in many ways. Some women are randy as can be during gestation (those lucky gals!) and their husbands are in man-heaven. Other women would sooner opt for a root canal than the insertion of their man's member into their birth canal. To make the picture even more complicated, men may have varied reactions when their, ahem, if I may say, sexy goddess blossoms into a Madonna. And I don't mean the one who vogues. So let's take this scenario by scenario.

Scenario #1: You want it. He's afraid he'll hurt the baby, or break the law, or go to hell.

Dr. Walsh says: Get him the necessary medical information to assuage his fears about safety. Get yourself an empire-waist nighty from Victoria's Secret, a black lace thong, and a pair of stilettos that will never see pavement. If all else fails, obtain a certificate of permission from his priest or rabbi.

Scenario #2: He wants it. Finds you a babe. You feel like a fat cow and couldn't possibly.

Dr. Walsh says: Close your eyes. Muster all the images you ever had of being slim and raring to go. And, no, it's not cheating to think of former lovers or movie stars. (Just don't call out their names.) If your problem is lubrication, try the myriad of commercial lubricants out there. They even sell them in grocery stores now. If painful intercourse is an issue, or if you feel dizzy lying on your back, try lying on your side and welcoming him from behind. If all else fails, use the lubricant on him. Remember, girl, corkscrew motion. I know you can be a good hostess.

Scenario #3: Nobody wants it, and you're afraid you're growing apart.

Dr. Walsh says: There are many forms of intimacy outside of sexual intimacy. Making time to just be together is important. Talking is a great way to maintain closeness. And affection takes on new meaning when both your hands are probing the contours of the little being that's growing inside. Snuggle in bed with his hands on your tummy, and you'll know why some people refer to children as "the glue" in a relationship. Above all, know that this is a phase and your sexual relationship will go through many incarnations during the long haul. Keep talking about it to keep it conscious between you both.

111

Scenario #4: You both want it. Nobody's making it to the office anymore

Dr. Walsh says: Oh, to have such problems. If you want to keep your girlfriends, don't brag about it.

One final note: remember, there is no better way to bring on labor than some nipple stimulation and an earth-shattering orgasm. Once you hit thirty-nine weeks, girlfriend, my advice is to go for it. Personal disclosure: When I was thirty-nine weeks with my second child, I had no intention to relive the FORTY-TWO-WEEK pregnancy with my first daughter. So, at thirty-nine weeks, on the advice of an obstetrician, we farmed our five-year-old out to friends, ordered some spicy Chinese food, and vowed to knock boots until the sun came up, if that's what it took. It didn't take that. A little nipple action, and I was on my way to the greatest orgasm of my life as my water broke simultaneously. Okay, so the bed was a bit messy, but the pleasure and excitement of laboring while loving is a memory I'll cherish forever.

—Wendy L. Walsh, PhD, author of The Conscious Woman's Guide to Dating, Mating, and Relating—for Life!

The guys at Being Dad gave us a guy's perspective on sex during pregnancy.

The big question about sex and pregnancy is, Is your man a can or a can not? We've interviewed hundreds of men around the world for our Being Dad films, and it doesn't matter what color, religion, or nationality they are; some men can have sex during pregnancy and some can't.

Many women have told us that when their man tells them they aren't interested or can't do it, they thought it was because he didn't find them attractive in their later stages of pregnancy.

On the contrary, most guys think their partner is divine while pregnant. So what are the real and legitimate reasons that some men struggle with sex during pregnancy—particularly late-stage pregnancy?

1. He's scared of tapping the baby on the head.

It is amazing that some guys still believe it's possible, but I'm reliably informed it's not.

2. He feels like someone else is in the room.

Sure, if it was Jessica Simpson he probably wouldn't be complaining, but when he feels like his child is in the room it's understandable that he might have some issues.

3. It's a girl.

Many guys who knew they were having a girl said it made them feel very awkward to be getting intimate with their daughter so close by.

4. Logistics

It can seem like a logistical nightmare to find the right position, so you may need to suggest how to best tackle the problem and the right angle of attack.

5. He's scared of hurting you.

Communication is the key here. Talk him through what's OK and what's not. For example, he shouldn't put his weight on your stomach, but having cushions at the ready is required. Assure him that it's not uncomfortable for you and that he's not going to hurt you if you're in the right position and are using the right amount of force.

6. He thinks that his semen may induce birth.

Well he's not so stupid after all, as semen does contain prostaglandins, which can kick-start the whole shebang. It is unlikely that intercourse would have an effect much before the due date, so once again assure him he's not going to have to perform a home birth minutes after you've got down and dirty.

7. He doesn't know that your orgasms are potentially going to be earth shattering.

It's possible that female orgasms can be intensified in late-stage pregnancy due to the general swelling and increased blood flow to the nether regions. He might just be interested to check that out for himself with some gentle persuasion.

8. He's forgotten that being intimate need not be just about intercourse.

There are plenty of ways that you can play around without having intercourse . . . maybe he needs a refresher course.

It would seem that there is a roughly even divide between men who have issues with sex during late-stage pregnancy and those who don't. Remember, if your man is struggling, it's most likely due to one of the reasons above and NOT because he doesn't think you are beautiful. Visit www.beingdadusa.com for more insight into the male mind.
　　　　　　　　　　—The guys at Being Dad

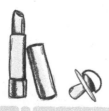

Bringing Your "Sexy Back"

Who says you have to wait until after the baby arrives to reclaim your sensuality? The first step to rekindling romance is to make sure you view yourself—with all your marvelous, new curves—as a woman who deserves attention. For many women, weight gain can have a huge impact on their self-esteem, and some pregnant mamas have to work harder than others at accepting their bodies. Confidence and lack of inhibition are always attractive to men, so as hard as it may be sometimes, really try and embrace your new figure and sexy curves.

Haven't you ever been in a room where a pregnant woman in full glow has captured all the glances? I can assure you that the men in the room weren't just appreciating motherhood; there were some serious looks going on. There's a certain sensuousness to pregnancy that reminds everyone of the joy of life, so take hold of your own curvy ride and realize your own beauty. As I mentioned before, you can dress up the curves, but don't just save it for "going out." Have fun on your nights at home together. In any case, before getting dressed, take a few moments to check out your naked body in a full-length mirror and say the following:

1. This body is truly amazing.

2. Every curve is a sensuous line.

3. My man cannot resist this gorgeous body.

4. I am a sexy Hot Mom goddess.

5. My breasts would make Pamela Anderson jealous!

Maternity Lingerie

Eve Alexander is the first line of exclusively maternity and nursing lingerie. Her babydoll set is designed to playfully curve your gorgeous belly ($33 at www.evealexander.com). Passion Spice also offers cute maternity camisoles and babydoll outfits ($29 to $34 at www.passionspice.com). What's nice about these camisoles is that they tie up the side or down the middle so they expand as your belly does, bringing you through the various stages of your pregnancy and adjusting and tightening to be worn or flaunted again after the baby is born!

The Reshape of Things

Your body is now changing in so many ways—focus on accentuating those sexy new curves. Your behind may have, um, expanded a bit, but your bosom most certainly has also. Having big boobs was one of my favorite perks of pregnancy. Growing up relatively flat-chested, there wasn't a push-up bra I hadn't met. It was so exciting the day I filled out a bra myself without the help of socks or tissues! I felt so womanly and feminine. It was a thrill—sore as they were, you couldn't catch me complaining! So accentuate and work your new assets! You know what brings out your sexy self. And so does he. Once you light the flares, the mood will shift.

Sharing Your Body

Once you've caught his attention—and believe me, he will notice—let your man participate in "helping" with your body. Start with a request for a head or foot massage. That's safe and feels good. Then you can encourage further exploration to the rest of your body. Let him know how good it feels to have him touch you. And you can reciprocate and enjoy.

Another fun way to increase intimacy is to let your honey shave your legs—yup, romantic and efficient, especially when your belly is making it a bit more difficult to see. Draw a warm bath and let him lather and shave your legs, turning a tedious task into a fun ritual. Just make sure he knows how to keep a delicate touch on your ankles. Also, it might be fun to get him to help with an impromptu toenail touch-up . . . with the fully truthful excuse that it's hard to see and reach that little baby toe.

There are other ways to get creative. Turn up the salsa or indipop for some exotic barefoot dancing, letting your curves tease his body. Write a love note with lipstick on your belly (you might want to use a washable ink pen!). Get him to help cook a fabulous meal with you in the kitchen: sharing the work, getting hot, and tasting off of fingertips can be very sexy. Maybe you can re-create one of your early date dinners. Once you see yourself as desirable and able, he'll sense that passion too, and you're sure to bring "sexy back."

A few words of caution: my husband had a very tough time getting past the idea that he would somehow hurt the baby if we had sex. Don't follow my example; jokingly saying "reassuring" things like "Don't worry, honey, it's not that big" does not go over well!

Rebirthing Your Relationship

Once you've awakened your sensual self and kick-started the romance, you'll feel empowered to make a few bold moves. No longer do you have to worry about getting pregnant, and if you have been "trying" for a while, then intimacy can become fun again, so let yourself enjoy the freedom. Also, I want you to know that this is definitely not just about sex. If you can continue the fun play of intimacy through pregnancy, it will make the post-birth relationship with your partner so much easier. Everyone has ebbs and flows of desire, but the trick to long-lasting couple success is to never let a dry spell go on too long.

One secret to keeping your sensual self and relationship in balance is TUA, or Time for Undivided Attention. This does not have to last for epic hours, but it must be a time when you both vow not to do other things. And it can't mean just plopping down on the couch to watch TV—you must be conscious and involved. Make it about discovery and understanding, sensuality and humor.

The point of this section is to help you feel more confident, not make you feel bad. If your pregnancy is high risk or you are so nauseous morning and night that sex is the last thing on your mind, it's OK. Sex is not the only way to create intimacy. You may be a couple that generally doesn't have an active sex life, and if it works for BOTH of you, then that's fine. Cuddling and watching TV or movies may be the way you enjoy spending your nights. I am not judging; it is all about what makes you two happy and satisfied.

Babymooning

You remember the honeymoon? By definition it is described as a holiday taken by newlyweds to celebrate their marriage and intimacy. Well, the rage these days is the "babymoon" . . . a time for partners to celebrate as a couple and relax on a getaway before the baby arrives. We went away for a weekend to Santa Barbara in my second trimester (the recommended time to go on your trip). Although I didn't realize I was going on a "babymoon" at the time, it was a fun trip and still holds great memories. If you can make this happen, by all means do. After the baby is born, a half-hour nap together feels like a vacation. Whether it's a hotel, a spa, a friend's cabin, a house-sit, or a beach, it doesn't really matter . . . it's just time for you to appreciate some peace away from all the ordinary interruptions. Many hotels and resorts now offer babymoons as another type of weekend package, with special perks and upgrades for expecting couples. My advice: make it simple so it's not about anything except you and your honey, relaxation, and the things you mutually enjoy. Just say no to baseball games, dance concerts, anything too strenuous, or a resort where a lot of partying and alcohol are present; it will only make you feel you are missing all of the fun. Avoid trips with too much transportation involved—taking connecting flights and then a small island hopper can make for a full day of travel and a lot of up and down air pressure. Talk to your doctor about flying. While many say it is safe until the third trimester, many recommend you stay on the ground if possible. So find out what is best for your body and condition, and for your own safety and sanity explore options like bed-and-breakfasts within driving distance first. Call the place you are thinking of staying and ask if they offer babymoon packages geared specifically for expecting couples.

This is not the trip for keeping a busy sightseeing schedule. Ironically, you might want to consider an adults-only resort; it will be much quieter and relaxing.

Ask if the place has twenty-four-hour room service (in case you get a 3:00 a.m. craving), and ask where the nearest hospital is in relation to the hotel. Be sure to pack lots of your favorite healthy snacks: this will help keep your blood sugar regulated and will make car rides and plane trips more enjoyable. If you are traveling out of the country, check to make sure your medical insurance covers you at your destination.

BUMP ON A BUDGET

If taking a pricey trip or time off work to go away just isn't practical right now, create a "babymoon" of your own.

- 🌸 House-sit for someone with a fabulous place, hopefully a friend or relative with a nice view and fireplace or a big pool (but stay away from the hot Jacuzzi). Being someplace new can feel fresh and exciting.

- 🌸 Create a "spa night" or weekend at home, filled with bubble baths and your favorite movie marathons. Relax with magazines and breakfast in bed (for you, of course), and commit to wearing your bathrobes all weekend. Turn off the cell phones and internet.

- 🌸 Have two massage therapists come to your home to give you both a "couples massage" (but make sure one specializes in prenatal massage).

❀ Do anything with sensuous, trancelike music: dinner, dancing, and romancing.

❀ Rent your favorite romantic movies.

❀ Look through all your couple photos. Take a journey through your relationship.

❀ Break out the sparkling cider and re-create as much as possible how you met and your initial flirtation: get into the role and let everyone wonder what's going on with the guy and that hot pregnant chick.

$TUFF TO DROOL OVER!

BabyMoon (www.baby-moon.eu) is a website dedicated to luxury hotels and resorts that offer babymoon accommodations. They provide a travel counselor who will recommend, research, and book your vacation. The St. Regis in California, for example, has a "Last Hurrah" package, which includes couples massages, a special cravings menu, discounts at baby stores in the area, fancy nonalcoholic drinks, and more starting at around $725 a night. The Four Seasons in Chicago has an "Expecting You" package, which includes body pillows, breakfast for two in bed, an in-room visit from the Ice Cream Man, a complimentary "Toast to Fatherhood" and cigar in the Seasons Bar for the expectant dad, complimentary pedicure for mom-to-be when she goes for her pregnancy massage, and discounts at local toy and children's stores, starting at approximately $460 a night. The Mandarin Oriental Hotel in New York offers a babymoon package that includes a welcome gift of sparkling cider and chocolate-dipped strawberries, an over-the-top gift basket of maternity lotions and potions, two hours of spa treatments for the expectant parents, and breakfast for two and a suite with a view. Rates fluctuate, but the package starts at $2,750 a night.

Vagina Push-Ups: AKA Kegels

The next time you pee, stop and squeeze midstream. The activity of squeezing and tightening your pelvic muscle is called a Kegel. Kegel exercises are the equivalent of push-ups for your vagina; they help get you in shape "down there," reinforcing the area for childbirth and *preventing you from peeing on yourself every time you sneeze or cough.* They also strengthen and tighten your pelvic muscles and area after birth. This is something your hubby will greatly appreciate. Now, I don't want to brag or anything, but I happen to be a Kegel professional. This was an activity in which I excelled. It made me feel so accomplished; I could complete two hundred of them a day without even breaking a sweat. They are so simple, and you can literally do them anywhere—at work, grocery shopping, while out to lunch, watching TV, or talking on the phone. In fact, I have been doing them the entire time I have been writing this paragraph!

Sex Put the Baby into You, and Sex Is Going to Help Get the Baby Out!

It is said that a natural way to induce labor is, you guessed it, having sex. Orgasms and nipple stimulation produce oxytocin, which causes the uterus to contract. Semen contains a hormone called prostaglandins (synthetic prostaglandins are given to women to induce labor), which also causes the uterus to contract and the cervix to soften. As with anything physical, always check with your physician!

Relationship Contractions

A pound of tired, a pinch of hormones, and a sprinkle of overwhelm is a recipe for stress on any relationship. As women, we are naturally maternal, and those instincts will kick in big-time once your baby arrives. Your current baby (aka your hubby) will be feeling the hit. There are lots of reasons why your relationship and sex life get more complicated after childbirth. Often, for a number of physical and hormonal reasons, some women lose their sex drive after birth, while lack of sleep can also contribute to a lack of interest in, or energy for, sex on both sides. Some men experience "delivery room

"My husband's idea of rough sex is when I don't shave my legs."
—Stephanie Blum, comedian and Hot Moms Club member

trauma," making it hard for them to see their wives as sexual beings . . . but most get over it in time . . . and your own drive will come back. I am telling you this so that you are aware and prepared if you and your hubby notice a difference in your sex life. Most women need emotional intimacy as a prelude or precursor to sex. For men, on the other hand, sex leads to emotional intimacy. So when the sex dries up, men tend to feel emotionally disconnected and may withdraw, and when he's withdrawn you may not feel the desire to be intimate, and so goes the vicious cycle.

There is no simple solution for everyone; you have to find what is going to fit for you two as a couple. However, being aware of the pitfalls many couples face after birth will help you navigate them. Being prepared and acknowledging that a healthy sex life is critical to a healthy relationship will help you prioritize working through it and communicating about it before delivery and afterwards.

Hot Mom Tips for Keeping the Spark Alive Post-Baby:

Praise and reward. Many moms in our club said they felt attracted to, and appreciative of, their husbands when they helped with housework and the needs of the baby. That made the moms-to-be more likely to be intimate with their husbands. The reward system, ladies: it never fails with animals, your kids, and your men. When they do something you like, praise, praise, praise.

If it's really something great, like cleaning the house and making you breakfast in bed, try your hardest to muster some "reward" that you think he would really enjoy. You know what that could be. Everyone likes to feel they have value in a relationship, and that they are good at something, so if your man wraps the best baby swaddle in town, tell him so and brag about it in front of others so he can hear. That pride will incentivise him to take on other tasks with the baby and doing things for you, which in turn will make you more attracted to him and excited to be intimate with him. Now THAT is the cycle you want to keep going!

Keep your relationship a priority. We all want to be good parents, and we all want to know and do everything possible to take the best care of our newborns, but it is equally important that we remember to direct some of that energy into taking care of and nurturing our relationships with our partners. It is important to bring the baby into YOUR loving relationship, making you all a unit, not the two of you directing your energy to the baby. That is a big difference, which is crucial in preserving your family unit. Remember you are doing this for the sake of your child/children; you are modeling relationships for them. Because their future relationships will most likely mirror yours, they deserve to be a part of that same loving union that brought them into the world.

Good ol' date night. I wish I had some fancy or unique spin on this, but the truth is that setting time at least once a week to go on a date or having quality one-on-one time together is important and has proven to work. I add that you are absolutely NOT allowed to talk about the baby during your date. No exceptions!

Fantasize and surprise. Fantasizing and surprising one another can cement bonds and create deeper intimacy. I know it seems impossible to be flirty when you are exhausted and busy feeding, and changing a newborn every few hours, but it only takes a minute to write an enticing note or to leave a sultry message on his phone or nightstand. Arousal and intimacy begin in the mind, and anticipation is a HUGE turn-on. It's not as hard as you think. Little things really do mean a lot and go a long way. Try sending him a sexy card in the mail. Write a love note and hide it in a book he's reading. Call him on the phone and sing a silly love song. Make up the words. Sing out of tune. It only takes a few minutes and will definitely put a smile on his face. Spritz just a tiny bit of your fragrance on his briefcase so he has the scent of you all day. Use your lipstick and leave him a sultry message on the bathroom mirror. Flash him a sweet and sexy smile when he least expects it, or just flash him for fun! Igniting the passion really is just as easy as touching him affectionately when you walk by or giving him a quick pat on the butt. Get creative! Come up with special code words for "I want you!" for when the kids or relatives are around. Instead of a peck on the cheek, surprise him with a sensual kiss as he heads out the door; it can literally change the course of the entire day. It really is the little things that build intimacy and ignite passion. Everyone wants to feel desired, even men.

Create a sacred space. Declare your bedroom a Toy-Free zone! As moms, our homes quickly become ridden with toy trucks, swings, and the latest activity mats. It is sooo important to keep at least one room—your bedroom—as your sacred space, your sanctuary.

It should be "husband and wife's" bedroom, not "Mom and Dad's" bedroom, if you know what I mean. It is hard to get physical if you have kids in the bed or if you are rolling on action figures. . . . It should be a room for making love, or just relaxing and reading together, or watching your favorite shows, a place for bonding and intimacy that doesn't involve the kids. Claim that space. Put candles and flowers by the bed. Have photos of the two of you as a couple. No family or baby pictures in this room—they can be anywhere and everywhere else in the house, but this room should be designed to inspire connection and romance. I know it sounds corny, but believe me, it works; our environment sets the mood and can easily turn us on or turn us off.

Feel sexy because you are sexy! A little lingerie can spice up your love life, especially after maternity underwear has become a staple. Lingerie is a turn-on for your man, but it should also make you feel feminine, womanly, and beautiful. If, like most new moms, you start to feel a little self-conscious about your body and are working to get things back to where they were pre-baby, I recommend babydoll dresses. They offer support up top and are loose fitting and very forgiving below. Keep in mind the fact that confidence is your sexiest weapon. Own that you are fabulous and a Hot Mom no matter what your new shape currently looks like. We are our own worst critics. The more comfortable you are with yourself, the sexier you will feel and the sexier you will be. Sexy doesn't have to mean lingerie; it's anything that helps you get in touch with the woman inside of you. It could be red lipstick, a manicure, or a hot bath to make you feel sensual. Sexy is an attitude and a feeling. It all starts with you. As a mom, your depth of loving and caring will be stronger than ever, so don't forget to turn a little of that love toward yourself!

Talk with your partner, commit to keeping the intimacy and making it an important priority. Start now; get a plan to keep your relationship on track once baby arrives. Communicate, work together, use the tips above, and remember that sharing a child together can cement a relationship and help bond you in ways you never imagined.

Okay, a lot of the things you've read about in this chapter I didn't do, but I wish I had. The truth is, I didn't see myself as sexy when I was pregnant, and that was my biggest mistake. I let my ideas of my old sexy self get in the way of finding power in my new developments. It was my self-esteem during pregnancy— not my cramps or aches—that was the biggest hurdle to regular intimacy. Remember, if you can realize that your body and sexuality are not only working but beautiful as well, you'll go a long way to keeping your relationship and happiness intact!

JOURNAL—MONTH SEVEN

1. Write down all the qualities that make you a beautiful, sexy woman—as you are right now, today!

_____

_____

_____

_____

_____

_____

_____

_____

_____

_____

_____

_____

_____

2. For fun, write a "naughty" story or fantasy you are having right now. (Give a copy to your man.)

_____

_____

_____

3. List all the things that make you feel sensual, smart, and sexy: foods, music, fabrics, literature, movies, jewelry, creative projects. Keep the list handy.

_____

_____

_____

_____

_____

_____

_____

_____

_____

_____

_____

_____

_____

_____

_____

_____

_____

_____

_____

4. What's the most romantic and sexy thing your man has done for you recently? What is the most romantic thing he could do post-baby? (Don't forget to hint that to him.)

_____

_____

_____

_____

_____

_____

_____

_____

_____

_____

_____

_____

_____

_____

_____

_____

_____

_____

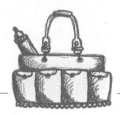

Eight

Milking It

During those nine months, it can seem like forever,
but after you have given birth, you realize
just how precious that time was—the incredible
connection between just the two of you.

—Nicole Delareta, mom of two and Hot Moms Club member

Pregnant women steal the attention—of course, you don't mean to, it's just that everyone else pales in comparison. Even if you can't see your own magnificence and glow, others do, and it will bring you gobs of attention, ready or not. Perfect strangers smile at you and ask what you are having. People you barely know will start conversations with you about birthing and parenting tips. Clerks and waiters become your best friends—and you get excellent service.

Anyone standing beside a pregnant woman becomes invisible—and trampled upon—as the world rushes in to help the mom-to-be. People will open doors for you, offer you their seat, let you cut in line, and carry any heavy object. Case in point: I gave birth in December and so was eight months pregnant during the holiday shopping season. I learned the wonderful secret that full-blown pregnant women get access to the employee bathroom, preferential treatment at checkout (in fact, a cashier even opened a line specifically for me), and help bringing the bags to the car! If only things were so civilized all the time. . . . The key is to rub your belly, put your hands on your back, and work up your most Oscar-winning angst look. That's right, *MILK IT!* There are only a few times in your life when you will get the star treatment, and the bigger the belly, the better it gets. . . . That's right, I said it, and I mean it—work the perks and the help of strangers because it diminishes pretty fast after the baby is born. During pregnancy, I'd have three people rushing to open the door for me. Afterward, when I was truly struggling to get the door open while balancing a newborn, a stroller, and a massive diaper bag, people walk right past never thinking to help. So bask while you can!

Kick, Kick, Hooray!

Your baby is going to be angling for some of the attention and spotlight as well. You may have noticed that your little one loves to kick and stretch. What started out as a little fluttering may feel like popcorn popping in your belly or a mini kickboxing class underway. I remember entertaining friends and neighbors with random body parts rolling across my belly or playfully tapping my bump and watching as the baby knocked back. Really enjoy and soak in these adorable moments; the kicking and punching is not nearly so cute or fun when your baby becomes a toddler!

The kickTrak is a device that helps you count the baby's kick patterns and frequency, helping you feel connected to and confident in her or his well-being. This can also be a fun way to help your other child or children bond with you and the baby by having them sit with you and keep track of the baby's kicks. You'll find the kickTrak at www.babykick.com.

The Ultimate Accessory

Fully pregnant during Halloween? Your belly is the ultimate costume accessory! Some of my favorite costume ideas are guaranteed to make a fun statement and have you be the talk of any bash. A few suggestions:

Water-based Belly Paint can be found at www.castingkeepsakes.com.

- ❀ Fishbowl: Paint a fish and bubbles on your belly and wear a light blue-and-white outfit.

- ❀ Speed "bump": Take a yellow sweat suit and run over it with the car (you may have to paint the tires to get a nice black mark). Toss it on and, voila, your belly is the "bump."

- ❀ Basketball player: Paint your belly orange and black, à la a basketball, and then dress in the outfit of your home team. For photos put your hands on your belly as if you are holding a ball.

🌸 Environmentalist: Paint the earth on your belly and wear *Save Our Planet* or any eco-statement clothing.

🌸 Crystal ball: Paint your belly in swirling mystery with blues and whites, dress in a gypsy costume, and rub your hands over your belly. Be sure to make fun and outrageous predictions to all the party guests. This works great also as a magic 8 ball.

If you are not comfortable exposing or painting your belly, try these fun alternatives:

🌸 "Miss Conception": Dress in a ball gown and make a "Miss Conception" sash à la a beauty pageant contestant. (This one is fun no matter what stage of pregnancy and could be an interesting way to tell everyone if you haven't announced it yet.)

🌸 Pregnant Grandma: We all know the pregnant nun costume—and your hubby can go as a priest. Here's another take that's also sure to win some laughs: go as a pregnant grandma, with gray wig and cane. Your man can go as your young stud! Sure to be a fun conversation starter!

Babe-with-a-Babe

Since Demi's famous photograph, women everywhere have started showing off their growing bellies and documenting their pregnancies in portrait photography. Today, moms are stronger, sexier, and more confident than ever. What better way to record this awesome new-mom glow than a photo session with a professional photographer? Who said you can't still be a babe when you are having a baby? A pregnancy photo shoot is the perfect way to prove it and the best excuse to feel like a supermodel for an afternoon. Your life has been changing from the minute you found out you're pregnant, and having a few good photos will boost your confidence and help you feel glamorous and desirable.

It's hard to believe, but in a few years, it will be difficult to remember how you felt during those last few weeks—a beautiful framed reminder can connect you back to these days. I recommend scheduling your photo shoot six to ten weeks before your due date, or eight to twelve weeks for multiple births. Your man and older children can make great additions to your session. If you are on the fence, I say do it; you might be pleasantly surprised at how amazing you can look and how special those photos will make you feel afterward. Once your little angel is born, you may regret not having done it.

Today, most photography studios have a pregnant mom package. This is one of the things I wish I had done, but ten years ago it was not common or easily accessible. So go for it! Channel that inner supermodel!

Feel Beautiful
Because You Are Beautiful:
How to Get the Perfect
Pregnancy Pictures and
Why This Is Such a Wonderful
and Emotional Event

I can't tell you how important it is to document those last few weeks of your pregnancy. Women today are embracing their growing bellies, and even if you might lack a little self-confidence, a photo shoot with a professional photographer can help you feel beautiful and sexy. Hire someone who specializes in maternity photography who will work within your comfort zone to capture just how beautiful pregnancy is. Experiment with different poses, props, fabrics, lighting, and angles to make you feel your best. Whether it is your first or last pregnancy, it is an experience you will never forget.

I've had the opportunity to photograph beautiful, pregnant bellies for over six years, and I love that I can help women embrace motherhood. Expecting a child is one of the most unbelievable feelings, and you should want to preserve that feeling. Your life changes from the minute you find out you're pregnant, and I believe that there is nothing more beautiful and amazing than an expecting mother.

Most pregnant women I have photographed feel so alive and strong—and they want to capture this newfound empowerment.

Remember, it's not just a photo shoot, it is an experience—one that you won't want to forget. And when you look back, it will be so much more than a photograph. The resulting portrait will be a piece of artwork to always remind you of your special nine months.

—Jessie Prezza,
maternity and baby photographer

Knowing that this may be my last pregnancy made it so important to capture the amazing life growing inside of me. Having photos taken was an outward expression of how beautiful and sexy I felt on the inside. I completely embraced the changes that my body was going through, and I felt sexy and strong. Capturing that splendor gave me photos that will be with us forever. During the shoot, my husband loved me more than ever and my four-year-old son, Jaden, treated me like a princess. I was the "vessel" carrying a part of all three of us. I can never get that feeling back, and there's nothing on earth that emulates the magnificence of the pregnant belly. When I'm seventy, I hope to look back on my beautiful pictures and remember what an awesome experience pregnancy was and what a Hot Mom I had been!

—Katie Hestla,
mom of two and Hot Moms Club member

Award-winning pregnancy photographer and Hot Moms Club favorite Jennifer Loomis (www.jenniferloomis.com) shares some of her tips and ideas with us on what to look for when researching a photographer to take your pictures.

"Having photographed women since 1993, I have had women come to me who were shy and uncertain about doing this. Afterwards not one of them regretted it, saying that their nine-month pregnancy was such a short time and that the photographs helped them see their beauty and feel good about the changes occurring in their bodies. But there is an added benefit. After photographing women for so long, I now have children who were once inside their mothers' pregnant bellies during the photo shoot, telling me how special it is for them to have those photographs. One client's daughter wanted the photographs of her inside her mommy's belly hung in her room so she could see the pictures as she would take her nap."

The average pregnancy photo shoot happens six to eight weeks from your due date, so there's almost no room for error if you don't like the finished result or the photographer makes a mistake. Here are five tips on how to make the best choices when selecting a pregnancy photographer:

1. **Look for experience.** The photographer should either have extensive experience in or specialize in pregnancy photography, in

order to obtain the most flattering poses for a pregnant woman's body.

2. **Consider artistry and personality.** Finding someone whose work you love and whom you want to work with is key to capturing beautiful images of your pregnancy. Also look for redundant images on the artist's website, which indicates a lack of creative artistry.

3. **Ask for referrals.** If you weren't personally referred by someone who has used the photographer and can recommend his or her work, ask for several referrals to contact. These may be already posted on the photographer's website.

4. **Start to finish.** Ask if the photographer will be thoroughly involved in the editing and photo selection process; this represents about one half of your cost. The photographer should expertly guide you to the best and most unique photos, plus offer suggestions for cropping and finishes.

5. **Get technical.** Ask if the photographer uses film or digital. I prefer film; darkroom prints have a superior archival quality over digital prints. Film is more expensive, but the quality and longevity are worth it, so you can pass the images down through the generations.

Once you have found the perfect photographer, here are some ways to make the most of your shoot. Relax, enjoy, get lost in the moment. The right photographer will know how to capture that and help put you at ease. It may take a few frames to get comfortable and into your groove; that is normal. Looking good on the outside helps you feel good on the inside—that is just a fact—and, conversely, when you feel good on the inside you want to reflect that in the way you present yourself. So glow, shine, and be gorgeous, get your hair cut or blown out before the shoot and splurge on getting your makeup professionally done. (Most photographers offer this as part of the package; if yours doesn't, have a stylish friend help or make an appointment at a makeup counter in an upscale department store.) Do whatever it is you normally do that makes you feel your most confident and glamorous. The last thing you want is to get the photos and think, *This is a great shot, but look at my split ends,* or *Yikes, my nails are all chipped. . . .* Don't worry if you have a breakout, the photographer can edit and smooth out your skin afterwards. Some women prefer to be shot by themselves, others like having their partner and/or other children in the photographs, and some opt for a mix of both. It's up to you. There is no right or wrong way, it is all preference and how you want to mark this moment in time. You may opt for a charming beach shoot with a peak and hint of exposed belly, or you may feel totally at ease in a studio completely in the buff in all your glory. Think about what you want and then do it! You can always toss the photos if you don't like them, but you can never go back and shoot once your baby is born.

The Shape of Things!

I know I keep encouraging you to celebrate your shape, and some of you may feel more like a Thanksgiving float than a sexy goddess, but when it's all over you will miss feeling the baby inside of you, and you will definitely forget how big you were. To preserve you in all of your glorious largeness, cast your belly. Imagine a full-scale, three-dimensional sculpture of your beautiful bump. You can do this yourself with plaster. Belly casting is another intimate and fun way to capture your pregnant image. It can be a sensual experience with your honey, or it can be a fun project to do with your older children. It's as simple as putting plaster on your belly or breasts, waiting until it's semidry, and voila! You have a cast that you can use as your canvas. Once it's totally dry (about twenty-four hours), use watercolors or acrylics to decorate your latest, greatest work of art. You can find fun suggestions for the painting process online: planets, faces, designs, names, flowers. You could save painting it until after the birth, and then use your little one's feet and hands as the decorative motif.

If they're reinforced and waterproofed, belly casts can also be used for flowers, a baby time capsule, or even a "baby bowl"—just line with blankets and your newborn can have a rest in a very familiar curve.

Belly Vita has Belly Imprint Spa Treatment and Sculpting Kits for the full experience (www.bellyvita.com).

I have a friend who made gorgeous bronze casts from the belly mold of each of her three children. She engraved their names, birthdays, and birth weight on the bottom of each one. She uses them as decorations in her home—one even sits on her dining room table as a fruit bowl!

To turn your belly into a true work of art, Bronze Bowls by Mamas Belly (www.mamasbelly.com) takes your belly cast and bronzes and engraves it.

For those special last few weeks, you may want to consider a henna tattoo for that fabulous belly. Henna (and other natural body paints) are perfectly safe, and what better canvas to use than your curving tummy? The complex designs of henna art require an artist with some skill, so you can also use watercolor body paint kits or temporary rub-on tattoos (tummy tats) in creating your belly art. If you have other young children, this can be an activity that the kids can join in on. It may not be great art, but what a fun and silly way to share in the expectations of a new baby. And just think, all these designs are like leaving a love note on your belly!

> "By far the most common craving of pregnant women is not to be pregnant."
> —Phyllis Diller

Visit www.proudbody.com for nontoxic belly-painting kits and www.doulashop.com for henna tattoos and tummy tats. My favorites? *Mommy+Daddy* and *Love at First Kick.*

Celebrate Your Pregnancy—or Not

You may be excited to become a parent, but at this point in your pregnancy, no matter what you try, you would rather wake up at sunrise, run ten miles, sit through an all-day board meeting, get a root canal, and then have dinner alone with your mother-in-law than be pregnant another day. You're not alone. You've read all the peppy books and you bought the trendy pregnancy clothes and all the fun baby gadgets, but you are just fed up with being pregnant, and you are counting the days, hours, and minutes until it is over!

> *"The best thing about pregnancy was birth."*
> —Jennie Goodwin, mom of two and Hot Moms Club member

I know many moms who love being a mom, but their bodies disagreed with pregnancy. If you are feeling this way, know that it's fine and nothing to be ashamed of. Many moms-to-be feel guilty that they don't love it or that their pregnancies don't mirror those of the actresses on TV smiling effortlessly with their bare bumps showing. If you feel you need a laugh or proof that you are not alone, visit www.sucksandthecity.com and read Joanne Kimes's hilarious book, *Pregnancy Sucks: What to Do When Your Miracle Makes You Miserable.*

House Arrest,
Commonly Known as Bed Rest

I was not sentenced to bed rest, but I have several friends who were. Ahhh, "bed rest." Sounds pleasant, right? Bed + Rest: having an actual excuse to be lazy should have you jumping for joy. Instead, after several days, most moms-to-be feel bored and uncomfortable from lying on one side or from lack of activity. It is going to be hard to sit idly by as your kids tear up the house or you watch your hubby butcher dinner. But try to take a few deep breaths and know that it is only temporary. As boring and frustrating as bed rest can be, keep reminding yourself that you are doing this for the health of your baby—the first of many sacrifices you will make for your children.

BED REST CHECKLIST

❀ Have your doctor outline specifically what you can and cannot do.

❀ Keep a phone nearby.

❀ Get a great robe and cozy jammies. (First and foremost you need to be comfortable, but keep in mind that friends and relatives may be stopping by often to see you, so opt for pajamas that are clean and comfy, but also cute. You will feel presentable rather than embarrassed.)

❀ Invest in a laptop or borrow one. You can connect with other moms on bed rest, shop for last-minute baby items, research, or work.

Club Bed

For moms on prolonged bed rest, a little pampering may be in order. There are great services that bring the spa right to your bed, such as Spa Where You Are (www.spawhereyouare.com) and Mobile Spa (www. mobilespa.com). Bed rest may feel like a jail sentence, so it is important to fill your days with things that help you feel accomplished instead of helpless, like finishing all the thank-you notes from your shower and engaging in uplifting activities like reading sassy mommy books that will make you laugh and get you psyched up about motherhood.

A FEW HOT MOMS CLUB FAVORITES

❀ *Sippy Cups Are Not for Chardonnay* and *Naptime Is the New Happy Hour* by Stefanie Wilder-Taylor

❀ *Notes from the Underbelly* and *Tales from the Crib* by Risa Green

❀ *Knocked Up* by Rebecca Eckler

❀ *Belly Laughs* by Jenny McCarthy

This is also a great time to start a meal delivery service or have that friend who is an amazing chef bring over a few home-cooked meals. Keep in mind that you can't run away. You are stuck in your spot, so as much as you'd love company, don't invite well-meaning, long-winded neighbors or friends over!

Another tip: remember that expensive baby monitor you got? Set it up so that you can talk (yell) at your kids or husband from any room in the house. Walkie-talkies are equally effective.

YOU KNOW YOU'RE OVER BED REST WHEN . . .

✿ Your eyes light up at the thought of going to your doctor appointments.

✿ You want to smack the next person who says, "I wish I was on bed rest" or "I would change places with you in a heartbeat."

✿ You haven't been this caught up on *Days of Our Lives* since college.

✿ You've called your husband fourteen times and crank-called your brother twice, and it's only noon.

✿ You've learned to speak Spanish, French, and Russian.

✿ You've knitted a hat for everyone you have ever met.

✿ You can now write perfectly with your left
   hand and can write your name legibly with
   your toes.

✿ You've finished all of your Christmas cards
   . . . and it's only June.

I know at times it may feel like a jail sentence, but try to relax and remember that it is only temporary—meditate, visualize, get caught up on all of those films and all those e-mails.

Sidelines National Support Network, founded in 1991, is an organization that helps moms-to-be cope with bed rest or high-risk pregnancies.

Party Time!

Some people live for baby showers, the corny games, the itty-bitty clothes, and the cuteness of it all. Others look forward to this as much as an appointment at the DMV. The hard fact is—whether you like it or not—you NEED a baby shower if this is your first baby. You will be amazed, astounded, and downright blown away at all of the baby things you have to have. My suggestion: tailor the party to your taste. Make sure the person planning the event knows whether you like games or not; whether to keep it short and sweet (if you haven't been feeling well); or whether you want the baby shower event of the year, soup to nuts. You can keep things traditional with gifts, cake, and games—or you can step outside the box and suggest a themed baby shower.

SOME GREAT BABY SHOWER THEME IDEAS

🌸 Throw a "Hot Mom" baby shower!

🌸 Baby book showers are becoming more and more popular. In addition to a gift, each guest brings her favorite childhood book with a note to the baby on the first few pages, so he or she and Mom will always remember who it came from.

🌸 Pamper Mommy shower is perfect for a second-time mom who already has many of the baby things. Get her spa trips, massages, a night of free babysitting, food service, etc.

🌸 This Is Your Life shower is another fun option. Everyone brings old photos of the mom-to-be and talks about her "before" and how much her life is going to change. Share funny stories and talk about the qualities she has that will make her a great mom.

🌸 Try a Noah's Ark theme shower for parents having twins—guests bring two of everything!

🌸 Throw a shower with an astrology theme. Gifts can tie into the mom's and baby's birthstone colors.

🌸 Time of the Day showers are supercreative and practical. Guests are assigned a specific time of day—breakfast, bath time, bedtime, playtime, etc.—and they are responsible for bringing baby items that could be used for that period.

✿ A Star Is Born baby shower is sure to make the mom-to-be feel like the star of the show. Create a red carpet, decorate in gold and silver, and have the guests dress in their glamorous best. Play "celebrity mom" guessing games. And for added fun you can go to the star registry and have a star named after the baby.

✿ Lil' Pumkin showers are perfect for those delivering in October.

✿ A Stay at Home Mommy shower is ideal for the mom on bed rest or the mom who is not feeling great. Hold a low-key get-together in the mom-to-be's home and have guests come in their robes and slippers.

✿ Host a Helping Hand shower if the mom-to-be has everything she could possibly need and more. Have a get-together to celebrate the mom and her new journey, but let the guests know that all of the gifts will be donated to a needy shelter for expecting moms or a specific single struggling mom.

Other Great Ways to Make Your Shower Memorable:

Two Plums Paper (www.twoplumspaper.com) has the most adorable adornments to complement any baby shower. Their birth blessings kits allow guests to connect and bless both mom and baby.

Scrapbooking has become more and more popular. Adding a scrapbooking station to any baby shower is the perfect way to pass off the baby album work to your friends and family! Plus they'll enjoy creating a page and being part of the memories to come. S.E.I. (www.shopsei.com) has the best selection of colorful yet very cool scrapbook pages.

Design-her Gals (www.designhergals.com) allows you to custom make stickers, notepads, and more to match the mom-to-be's look. These work as a personal and fun touch, or as a great party favor.

Glasses filled with M&M's make delicious centerpieces and guest gifts. Customize them with the baby's name or funny sayings. Visit www.mymms.com for ideas.

The Baby Bunch (www.babybunch.com) creates adorable bouquets made from baby clothes, socks, and hats. They double as a centerpiece and a gift.

Baby Diaper Cakes (www.bloomersbaby.com) also make popular and fun centerpieces.

A fun shower gift for a couple is the "It's Your Turn" reversible pillowcase set. One side says *On Duty,* the other side says *Off Duty* ($32 at www.uncommongoods.com).

Create a giant work of loving art. I was at a baby shower recently where there was a giant canvas, portioned off in shapes with masking tape, and fun colors and paintbrushes. Guests were asked to paint a section for the baby. As someone with no artistic ability whatsoever, I was a little reluctant for fear I would ruin it, but I found it fun and just made my small spot abstract and colorful. When it dried, they peeled off the tape and it truly was a gorgeous collage.

THE MOST BEARABLE BABY SHOWER GAMES AND ACTIVITIES

✿ *Baby Needs a Name Game.* If they haven't decided, help them out. Take a blank piece of paper with all of the alphabet letters from A to Z written on it. Photocopy one for each guest. Hit the timer. Everyone has two minutes to write down her favorite name for each letter.

✿ *Guess the Baby.* Every guest brings a baby picture. The person to guess the most pictures is the winner.

✿ *The Price Is Right.* Purchase several random baby items and have the guests write down the price of each item without going over. The winner gets a prize.

✿ *Are You an Artist?* Everyone gets a paper plate and a pen and puts her initials on one side of the plate, then flips the plate over and places it on top of her head. Guests have one minute to draw a picture of a baby. When they are done, they give them to the mom-to-be to hold up and pick her favorite.

❀ *Baby Bank.* Ask guests to bring some spare change and pass around a piggy bank for the baby. As each guest puts in some change, she has to give the mom-to-be some of her best advice. Ha!

Why Not Shower with Men?!?

Dads are more involved than ever in the parenting process. Co-ed baby showers including dads are becoming increasingly popular—it's more like a party. Some important rules, though: invite more than two guys, have the shower on a "non-game day," and get prizes that guys would like—a case of beer, gag gifts, etc.

Spin the Baby Bottle

FUN GAMES THAT GUYS MIGHT LIKE

❀ *Baby Jeopardy.* Test your baby knowledge. Break into table teams or guys against the girls. Make up your own trivia or buy pre-made baby jeopardy games.

❀ *Diaper Olympics.* Relay-race style . . . see how fast the guests can diaper a baby doll.

❀ *Bottle-Sucking Contest.* This is a lot harder than it looks and takes a long time, so I suggest filling the bottles only a quarter of the way. (For the men, fill the bottles up with beer!)

❀ *Name That Tune.* Make a CD of all songs with *baby* in the title, play a few lines, and let the guests guess.

❀ *Name the Baby Food.* Blindfold the guests and let them taste several jars of baby foods (you will be surprised how wrong they will be!).

❀ *Make a Baby Game.* Pair off guests (one guy and one girl) with play dough or markers. The team has one minute to "make a baby." The expectant couple picks its favorite, and that team wins the prize.

❀ *Tell All.* Everyone writes down a funny child-hood story anonymously. The parents-to-be read them out loud and try to guess the author!

Who needs a shower? Throw a Red Egg and Ginger Party! It's a Chinese tradition to hold a celebration one month after the baby is born to introduce the little one to friends and family. Hard-boiled eggs are dyed red and given to the guests, as the color red symbolizes luck and happiness and eggs represent fertility and the renewal of life. The Chinese feel ginger is important because the yin (cold) and yang (hot) balance their food and the ginger adds hotness to a tired new mother's nutrition because she is too weak (cold) from giving birth.

In Japan, they do not do showers; it is customary to give gifts after the baby is born. They believe the dog is the symbol of good fortune during the baby's birth, as it is believed to give safe and easy deliveries. So for fun, get a dog stuffed animal and bring it with you to the hospital or birthing center. (It can't hurt!)

BUMP ON A BUDGET

Register for your baby shower at Target (www.target. com). They have a huge selection of great items for less, so dollars go further!

ECO-MINDED MAMA

www.giggle.com, www.babyearth.com, www.naturally trendy.com, www.thelittleseed.com, www.theultimate greenstore.com, and www.newbornmom.com are a few great eco-friendly sites on which to register for your baby shower. The Right Start also offers an eco-friendly selection (www.rightstart.com).

For a fun paperless invite, create a video-evite. Use your webcam or video camera to record a quick message to friends with the information on the shower. (This works when the shower is not a surprise of course!)

www.pingg.com has the most beautiful and stylish online announcements and invites!

Bel Bambini is the go-to shop for A-list Hollywood moms. Their online registry offers a majority of the items they have in their Beverly Hills boutique, including lavish yet fun stuff like a hand-painted prince and princess potty with toilet paper and a magazine holder for $125 (www.bel-bambini.com).

JOURNAL—MONTH EIGHT

1. How was that baby shower? Make sure you mention all the highlights and quotes from the people who were there.

_____

_____

_____

_____

_____

_____

_____

_____

_____

_____

_____

_____

_____

_____

_____

_____

_____

_____

2. Did you do the photo shoot? If so, how did it make you feel and what is your favorite photo? If not, why? What is holding you back?

_____

_____

_____

_____

_____

_____

_____

_____

_____

_____

_____

_____

_____

_____

_____

_____

_____

_____

3. What are your celebratory feelings right now? Also, because we're not all full of joy and light all the time, what are your tears and worries? Call and share these with someone you trust.

_____

_____

_____

_____

_____

_____

_____

_____

_____

_____

_____

_____

_____

_____

_____

_____

_____

_____

_____

4. Make designs for your belly-casting or tummy-painting session. Now, go out and get the materials, do the deed, and paste a picture here.

_____

_____

_____

_____

_____

_____

_____

_____

_____

_____

_____

_____

_____

_____

_____

_____

_____

_____

_____

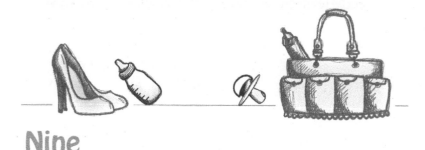

Nine

Expect-ations

This is it! The final month! The fat lady is just about to sing (or, in this case, scream in pain). It is obvious there isn't room for the both of you, and one of you has to go.
—Joanne Kimes, author of *Pregnancy Sucks*

The big event is just around the corner, and there's little else you can do but dream about the days to come. You have been planning and thinking about this baby for nine months. You may have planned for him or her for even longer—years of envisioning a son at Little League or a daughter at dance class (wearing those little pink tutus you wish you could still wear) or your little boy at hip-hop class and your little girl at soccer practice.

You've planned the baby's room and imagined her or his future . . . computer whiz, neurosurgeon, Stanford valedictorian, Madame President. . . . Whoa—don't get carried away! Keep in mind that it's a baby coming, a baby with its own plan and destiny to fulfill. You can shape babies, shower them with love and guidance, and protect them as much as possible, but they'll still have their own minds and be part of an entirely different generation. In today's changing times, your boy may hate cars or your little ballerina may love slimy worms and football.

The one guarantee is that your child will surprise you at some point, so developing an open mind now can mean happiness for all involved. But first things first—you still have one more month plus the journey of labor and delivery to deal with before you shape your child's destiny!

Ready or Not, Here She or He Comes!

For the last eight months, *you* have been doing all the prep work, mentally and physically. Now it's time to make sure the rest of the family is ready for the new arrival. A new baby can be a tough adjustment for any pets, siblings, and even your man.

Preparing Your Pet

Pets are extremely sensitive to smells and noises. There are certain scents and sounds that your pet perceives as "normal." The sound of a baby crying or screaming can be very stressful and scary for a pet that is not expecting it. There are CDs available that have the sounds of babies cooing, crying, laughing, and screaming—these are good to play in the months and weeks leading up to the birth to get your animals accustomed. (Go to www. dogmeetbaby.com for some great CDs.) Since dogs use their acute sense of smell to gather information, buy a generic new blanket and wrap the baby in it while in the hospital, then have your hubby bring the blanket home so your pets can get used to the baby's scent and "meet" before you bring the baby home. It is important that your pet respects and recognizes the baby as another "pack leader." Check with your vet or local animal trainer for the best techniques for your particular pet's personality.

Some helpful resources: *And Baby Makes Four: A Trimester-by-Trimester Guide to a Baby-Friendly Dog* by Penny Scott-Fox and *Cesar's Way: The Natural, Everyday Guide to Understanding and Correcting Common Dog Problems* by Cesar Milan, which has a section about preparing your dog for a new baby's arrival.

"Big Brother" Is Watching You

Whether your other children are three or thirteen, there is going to be some stress and adjustment to having a new sibling. They are used to having your undivided attention; the more you prepare them, the less chance you will have of aggression (acting out) or regression (acting more like a baby). Having a new sibling may be one of the biggest challenges for an older child, but it can also be the greatest gift.

Help your kids transition into the role of big brother or big sister by giving them a sense of pride. There are many companies that sell adorable *I'm a Big Brother* or *World's Best Big Sister* items, drawing attention to their new title and prompting others to strike up conversations with them about it. The more your children talk about it, the more comfortable they will be sliding into the role. Give your little one(s) responsibilities, like calling the grandparents once the baby is born and making the announcement. Assigning them any task involving caring for the baby will help them feel like you are working together as a team. Asking them to hand you diaper powder or assist in bathing the baby will help children feel important to you and to the process. Ask them to teach the baby things that the baby will learn anyway, like "teaching the baby to smile or laugh." When the baby does, they will feel like they are responsible—this will really help connect them to the child.

Many hospitals and birthing centers now take a family approach, offering sibling tours and classes. The more prepared he or she is, the more confident your child will feel.

Have kids make presents for the baby. Cards and drawings will help build the excitement and will make great keepsakes. Make sure you have a present from the baby to your other child or children—something they have been wanting, with a little note from the new arrival.

There are many great picture books that introduce the concept of "big brother" and "big sister" for children under five. Browse your local bookstore to find the one you feel your little girl or guy will most connect with. *Where Did I Come From?* by Peter Mayle (a classic) and *It's Not the Stork!* by Robie H. Harris are great books to guide children over seven who are asking questions and are capable of understanding more specifics about the process.

Nesting, aka Rearranging Things Over and Over Again for No Logical Reason

I never would have believed that anything, *anything* would make me spontaneously clean my house. But sure enough, the phenomenon of "nesting" is real. Now, it sounds all sweet and maternal, like a mama bird preparing her nest for her baby, but what I—and many moms I know—have come to realize is that nesting is this strange impulse to "organize."

I'm not talking about the need to "straighten up the house a little bit" because your friends are coming over; I'm talking about a strong, borderline-neurotic desire to color-coordinate the baby's outfits, or fold and refold the towels over and over until the corners line up, or change every lightbulb in the house for fear that one might burn out after the baby arrives. As the need to arrange and tidy takes you over, be sure to make and freeze a bunch of meals. You will be so glad after the baby is born, when you'll have no interest in cooking!

I Vant to Bank Your Blood!

Banking your baby's cord blood is all the buzz these days. I had never even heard of this when I was pregnant with my son ten years ago, but today you can't open a pregnancy magazine without seeing an ad about it, and many of the ob-gyns I have spoken with say they are constantly being asked their opinion on the subject.

Cord blood is the blood that is left in the umbilical cord after the baby has been born and the cord has been cut. For a long time it was tossed away, but scientists have discovered that your baby's umbilical cord blood is rich in stem cells, cells that can regenerate into most human cells. Studies show there are over seventy diseases that have been successfully treated using these cord blood stem cells.

If you decide this is something you would like to do, directly after the baby is born and the umbilical cord is clamped and cut, up to four ounces of blood from the placenta is extracted. It has no effect on the birth experience for you or your child, and there is no pain or danger to the mom or the baby by collecting the sample. However, it is advised that cord blood not be gathered in complicated or high-risk deliveries or interfere in the timing of cord clamping. Once collected, the blood is put into a vial or bag and sent to a storing facility to be frozen.

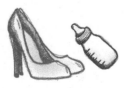

Public vs. Private,
and I Ain't Talking about Preschool!

Though private storage is expensive (it costs between $1,000 and $2,000 initially and then between $100 and $200 a year), the blood is reserved exclusively for your child or family members. The cord blood is stored and preserved in liquid nitrogen, and tests conclude that cord blood cells stored for fifteen years have the same composition as they did at the time of storage. Evidence suggests the cells should remain viable indefinitely if stored properly. Many parents feel it is biological insurance and potential protection for their child's future. There are many current uses and with advancements in science expanding and growing, the future potential use in regeneration is worth considering. This is literally a once-in-a-lifetime opportunity, as the cord blood cells can only be collected at birth. Private cord blood banking has become big business in recent years, and many medical groups feel they prey to some extent on parents' paranoia and fear. There is some debate, and more studies are being done, but research has found that your child's chances of needing the blood or being able to use *their own* blood is small—only 1 in 2,700. Now if your family has a history of sickle-cell anemia, leukemia, or other blood diseases, banking the cord blood seems like a smart idea, and your insurance company may even help cover some of the costs. Doctors warn there are no guarantees, however; if a child develops certain genetic diseases, his own cord blood is not going to be helpful, as it would contain the same genetic defects. Ultimately, if you can afford to do it, there is really no downside.

Many medical groups encourage parents to give the blood to public banks because the stem cells are more likely to be used this way. Keep in mind you cannot get the cord blood back if your child should later need it. But it's free; the cord bank pays for the collection and storage. About four to six weeks before your due date, contact a blood bank in your area or one affiliated with your hospital (www.marrow.org has a list of all participating hospitals in your state). They will give you a collection kit and paperwork to fill out prior to delivery. And while it is becoming more popular, unfortunately it is not available in all hospitals yet. If donating or banking your baby's cord blood is something you feel passionate about, or you want to learn more about the process and how you could help others, visit www.cordblood.com; 1-888-932-6568). They are the leaders in umbilical cord blood collection.

Whatever you decide, do your research, and be sure to talk it over with your doctor. Remember you are a good, caring parent regardless of whether you decide to store it privately for your own potential use, donate the blood, or forget the whole thing entirely.

Pack It Up

That precious due date has been on the calendar since your first visit to the doctor, and too often we count on that day as if it will really be the day. Today, there is a growing trend to schedule C-sections. Many of the moms I know plan their births like they plan a hair appointment. But if you're going vaginal, it's more than likely you will have an early arrival or a delayed departure. So don't panic if it's a week past your due date. And be prepared a few weeks before, just in case. If you are planning to give birth in a hospital or birthing center, you will need to pack a suitcase so you can feel as comfortable and relaxed as possible.

"FEEL GOOD" MUST-HAVES TO PACK

❁ Favorite pillow from home

❁ Cozy robe

❁ Slippers

❁ Extra socks (buy a new package of thick comfy ones)

❁ Comfortable panties (preferably briefs) and panty liners

    ❁ OnGossamer (www.ongossamer.com) has indestructible panties

    ❁ Belly Bandit (www.bellybandit.com)

Along with your "Feel Good" stuff, throw in a few "Look Good" items as well. Remember, you may be in many photographs and may have many visitors during your hospital stay. Be prepared for any photo op.

Make sure you pack your own camera and an extra disposable one. (It's important to have this just in case your camera runs out of batteries or the shutter breaks—this has happened to people I know, so always carry a spare!)

If you can't stand the thought of your first baby photos being taken with you in a drab hospital-issued delivery gown, bring your own! (Check out BYOG, Bring Your Own Gown, www.shopbyog.com and www.girliegowns. com for some comfy, pretty delivery gowns.) Also remember the following: makeup, travel sizes of your shampoo and conditioner, toothbrush and toothpaste, deodorant, travel razor, hairbrush, and lip balm or ChapStick.

Things you will thank me for reminding you about: your favorite power bars, crackers, and bottled juice and water; breath mints (you are going to have lots of visitors); your address book with all of the phone numbers of people you might want to call. Most hospital rooms even have wireless internet in your rooms so you can bring your laptop along.

For the Baby

You'll need to pack a new outfit or two. Choose something that is easy to slip on, with snaps in the front. (It's a little tricky slipping a onesie over a newborn's head.) Also, grab something with soft pants to ride home in, as the seat belt will fasten between the baby's legs. Depending on the season and climate, bring a blanket, hat, socks, or footsies. And don't forget the car seat. You won't be allowed to take the baby home without one. Many infant car seats offer extra head and body support. For those that don't, the Kiddopotamus Snuzzler provides the baby comfort and stability.

Presents

A few weeks before you are set to deliver, wrap a present for your older child or children, especially if that child will be visiting the hospital. This gift for them from "the baby" will be ready and waiting. Also, give her or him a disposable camera to take photos of the baby from the new older sister or brother's point of view. You may also want to bring a sentimental present for the new daddy or first-time grandparents, and I recommend picking up a few boxes of candy or some treat for the nurses taking care of you. It is amazing how far this gesture goes and how much nicer and faster your service is.

A charm bracelet or necklace is the perfect gift for a new mom. If your guy is well-meaning but isn't the type to think of this on his own, this might be a good time to start dropping some hints . . . and if this page happens to magically fall out of the book and land on your man's nightstand or in between the pages of his *Sports Illustrated*, well . . .

Push Presents

As if coming home with a healthy baby isn't enough, "push presents" are all the rage in Hollywood. Marc Anthony is said to have given Jennifer Lopez an eight-carat canary diamond ring after the birth of their twins, and Tom Cruise gave Katie Holmes a pair of pink-and-white diamond earrings when Suri was born.

Now, before you start rolling your eyes, there is actually something very sweet behind all the over-the-top bling. Having a sentimental gift or piece of jewelry to commemorate the birth of your baby is a lovely idea and well deserved after nine months of pregnancy and Xteen hours of labor. Although some celebrity couples take push presents to the extreme, yours doesn't have to break the bank to be amazing! Push presents should be something personal, something you will cherish and keep to remind you of that special day.

A charm bracelet is a popular gift; you can add charms with each new addition to the family. Or consider a charm necklace with a pendant or dog tag on which you engrave the baby's name and birthday. Fortunately there are so many companies out there that offer a variety of styles in every price range. Now, most guys will not think of this on their own, so it's time to start dropping hints by talking about the push present your friend just got, or mention something to his sister or mother.

$TUFF TO DROOL OVER!

Brooke Sheen loves her Heather B. Moore personalized charm collection (www.heathermoorejewelry.com). You can customize your own necklace, bracelet, or cuff links for dad. Necklaces start around $500 and up from there.

Jennifer Fisher Jewelry (www.jenniferfisherjewelry.com) offers the Charlotte Mom and Baby Necklace as seen on Kristin Davis in the movie *Sex in the City*.

Prices vary, but the average starts at $500. The Madison "Mom" Eternity Circle is also a head turner.

Nicole Richie was spotted everywhere with her stunning gold and diamond H necklace, for her daughter Harlow ($1,250 at www.jennifermeyerjewelry.com).

Trista Sutter received a Tacori Circle of Life Pendant, a classic necklace with inverted interior crescents representing the twelve months of the year. A diamond is placed into the month your baby is born (starting at $1,290 at www.tacori.com).

BUMP ON A BUDGET

Lisa Leonard Custom Necklaces are stunning and she has options starting at $40 and a big selection under $60 (www.lisaleonardonline.com).

Planet Jill has a big selection of photo jewelry and photo necklaces you can personalize (starting at $65 at www.planetjill.com).

Michele Baratta (www.michelebaratta.com) has the cutest variety of "brag" necklaces for under $75.

Sparkle Mom (www.sparklemom.com) offers affordable customizable birthstone jewelry, such as earrings, necklaces, rings, and bracelets.

ECO-MINDED MAMA

At Heart & Stone (www.heartandstonejewelry.com), fine silver engraved rivet rings are perfect for stacking with each new arrival. Made from 100 percent recycled silver. They also have gorgeous customizable dog tags and pendants.

The jewelry at Sentimental Silver (www.sentimental silver.com) is completely handmade, and the artist uses recycled silver.

Two Celebrity Favorites That Are Within Your Budget

Brooke Shields loves her customized Marnie Rocks birthstone necklace (www.marnierocks.com), and Jada Pinkett Smith wears a Robyn Rhodes custom birth necklace (www.robynrhodes.com).

Unique Items

Citrus Silver (www.citrussilver.com) takes engraved pendants to a whole new level, with unique shapes and designs.

Think about a mother and child ring from Penelope Poet (www.penelopepoet.com).

Camille Cesari's LovePrints (www.camillecesari. com) are gorgeous, handcrafted fingerprint jewelry. Each piece is a custom-made, unique work of art made of soft wax then cast in precious metal, harnessing your baby's fingerprint impression. The classic design is sure to be a great conversation piece.

Where Is That Stork
When You Need Him?

Preparing for the Big Day

By now you may have heard a lot about a "birth plan." This is simply an outline of how your ideal birth scenario would go. It's important that your doctor be aware of your desires. I am all for outlining your wishes and working toward making them a reality, but just be prepared that things don't always go as planned. You don't know how your body is going to react—if the baby will be breech or simply not want to come out. Everybody is different, and every birth you have may be different. Keep in mind that a successful birth results in a healthy mom and baby. Period. Whether you want an epidural, hospital birth, water birth, or natural, get all the facts, do your research, know your options, and talk to your doctor and other moms. Don't let anyone discourage you or encourage you to go against your instincts. But don't be afraid or upset if you have to change course. Have your plan, envision what you would like, but keep an open mind.

I gave birth in a hospital. I had the epidural and delivered vaginally after seven pushes. There wasn't time for a whole lot of fuss, decision making, or back rubbing; my son came quickly after labor started. I was young; I didn't have a birth plan; I just went to the hospital, did what I was told, and came home the next day with a healthy baby boy. I went to Lamaze class because that what was I had seen on TV; I wasn't as informed of my options as I am now. I have no regrets. My son is healthy, and truly that is the only result that matters.

Would I do things differently next time around? Maybe. Do I judge any mom for choosing a natural birth or a planned C-section? Absolutely not. You have to do what is best for you and what makes you feel most comfortable. Do your research, get all the facts, and ask your friends and relatives what worked best for them.

The ultimate goal is to feel confident and prepared for your big day.

Speaking of Being Prepared: Preregister

Call your doctor or hospital and talk to them about the preregistration process, many will encourage you to fill out all of your paperwork and consent forms a few weeks before the big day. The last thing you will want to do as you breathe in and out of contractions is fiddle with insurance information. I wish I had known of this option. I arrived at the hospital six centimeters dialated, and delivered less than two hours later. I vividly remember signing paperwork while I was in pain; I am not sure I even knew what I was signing, I would have signed just about anything at that moment. So if you can, preregister.

www.organizedfromthestart.com sells the Baby Briefcase, an organizer for all of your baby's important papers like the birth certificate, social security card, immunization records, and more. If you have a safety deposit box, make copies for the Baby Briefcase and keep the originals in the safety deposit box.

UNBELIEVABLE BIRTH FACTS!!!

❀ In 2009, the world's first surviving octuplets were born in Los Angeles, California, to Nadia Suleman. Known as "Octomom," this controversial single mom also had six other children under the age of seven.

❀ The Duggars from Arkansas gave birth to their eighteenth child in 2009. With only one set of twins, they had a baby pretty much every year since 1988. All of the children's names begin with the letter J!

❀ The smallest surviving preterm baby was Amillia Sonja Taylor, born October 24, 2006, at twenty-one weeks. Six days after delivery, she weighed only ten ounces. (Full-term births are thirty-seven to forty weeks.)

❀ The world's oldest mom, Rajo Devi, gave birth in India at the age of seventy. It was her first child.

❀ Jennifer Hoenig delivered twins on different days in different years. Her daughter arrived at 11:58 p.m. on December 31, 2006, and her son arrived just after midnight on January 1, 2007.

❀ Jayne Bleackley holds the record for the shortest interval between births—just 208 days—giving birth to a son on September 3, 1999, and a daughter on March 30, 2000.

✿ Elizabeth Ann Buttle holds the record for the longest interval between births—41 years—giving birth in 1956 and again in 1997.

Labor of Love

For fathers, *The Man's Guide to Labor and Delivery* is a straightforward yet funny video from DadLabs (www. dadlabs.com) that explains in detail what dads-to-be can expect during the labor and delivery process.

Around the time your wife is eight months pregnant, it will be suggested childbirth classes are in order. Let me rephrase that: You will be told to get in the car and go with your wife and get to childbirth class. My advice to you: Don't fight it. Aside from the breathing nonsense, you'll get to watch videos of an actual childbirth at childbirth class. No doubt you have seen a few Hollywood movies where an actress like Jennifer Aniston is covered in fake sweat but her lipstick remains perfectly intact, she starts screaming like the baby is eating

> her from the inside, and within five minutes
> a baby pops out covered in grape jelly, look-
> ing like a flawlessly formed and healthy six-
> month-old . . . so you're thinking, OK, I can
> handle that. . . . First of all, the childbirth vid-
> eo quality is second only to a Russ Meyer film
> taped in his garage. The lighting is bad, the
> camera jumps around, and there isn't Jenni-
> fer Aniston in sight. Hell, there isn't even John
> Aniston in sight. . . . Brace yourself.
>
> —Michael Crider,
> **author of *The Guy's Guide to***
> ***Surviving Pregnancy, Childbirth,***
> ***and the First Year of Fatherhood***

There are several respected birthing classes and methods to help you prepare for your childbirth.

Lamaze: "Learning to Breathe"

Maybe just as important as the techniques they teach you are the friends you meet. Lamaze class is a great place to "pick up" other couples with babies the same age. In summary, we saw a few graphic videos, learned a few breathing techniques, and got a bunch of numbers. I am not sure how much we used the techniques we learned—the whole delivery went rather quickly—but going to Lamaze class each week helped me feel as though I was getting more prepared. They answered lots of our questions and introduced me to some friends that my son and I still see, even eight years later.

Our first class we were running late, and after jumping—OK, rolling—into the car, I realized we had forgotten the pillow; my husband ran back in to grab one. It wasn't until we were walking into class that I realized he grabbed his Chicago Bears pillow that he has had since high school. It was worn and had traces of dog hair all over it. I asked him why he hadn't taken one of our nice pillows from the bed, and he said this one was in the hall cabinet and he didn't want to dirty a good one. Men! They don't realize that in Lamaze, your pillow reveals as much about you as your handbag or car, so make sure you have a comfortable one that is also clean!

Visit www.lamaze.org for information, or call the Lamaze International Hotline (800) 368-4404 about their philosophy and classes near you.

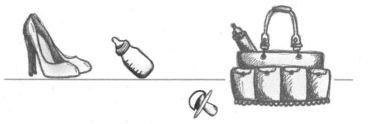

The Bradley Method: "No Spectator Sport"

The Bradley Method is a very comprehensive guide to delivery. It's a twelve-week course equally prepping the mom-to-be and focusing on the coach's role during the birth. Bradley sees birth as a bonding experience for families and fosters the end goal of natural childbirth by bringing dad off the sideline and into the game, teaching him relaxation and calming techniques, as well as birth positions. They also do labor rehearsals. Bradley provides small classes for maximum attention per couple and a 125-page workbook. There is no doubt you will be fully prepared! Now, you may lose your husband at the 125-page workbook and three months of classes, but to see if this is a fit for you, visit www.bradleybirth.com.

The Mongan Method—HypnoBirthing: "Taking the Birthing World by Calm"

This technique has become increasingly popular. It prepares both the body and the mind for a birth experience void of fear, pain, or tension. As we all know, the mind is powerful. This technique is said to help you eliminate your fears and harness that power within. The goal is to navigate the birthing process through preparation, visualization, and deep-breathing techniques. In theory I love this and am fascinated by the prospect, but would I be Zen enough to make it happen? For more information, visit www.hypnobirthing.com and read *Hypno-Birthing, The Mongan Method* by Marie F. Mongan M.Ed, M.Hy.

Belly Dance the Baby Out?!: "It's All in the Hips."

Today the ancient moves of belly dancing are being rediscovered and incorporated in many labor prep courses. Belly dancing was originally a fertility dance or birth dance celebrating pregnancy and women—it is the original form of labor preparation, as many of the moves are the same that the body naturally needs to deliver the baby. Belly dancing not only helps you move your hips and body during pregnancy but it also empowers you and builds confidence. Always ask your doctor if belly dancing is the right prenatal exercise for you, and always work with a trained belly dancing instructor.

Many belly dancing studios now offer pre- and postnatal belly dancing classes. It's a fun way to connect in a sensual way to your ever-changing shape, and you'll rehearse your muscles and hips—many of the moves mirror those needed in labor—while building your self-esteem!

Just as there are many different types of birth preparation classes, there are also several different ways and places to give birth, hospitals being the most common in the United States.

Water Birthing: H2 Oh Baby!

Water has a relaxing and calming effect on people. The thought behind a water birth is to provide a relaxed and calming atmosphere for both mother and child. Transitioning from the womb to an intimate warm birthing tub of water is supposed to be gentler on the newborn. To learn more details, check out www.waterbirth.org and *Water Baby: The Experience of Water Birth,* a video with footage from real water births and information all about it.

A-B-C-Section

As I mentioned earlier, there is a growing trend to schedule C-sections (30 percent of all U.S. births are now delivered by C-section). Some women are comfortable with this. I know others who would rather give birth in a dirty, crowded subway than have a C-section. Personally, I am neither for nor against elective C-sections, though the debate seems to be escalating. The goal here is to help you in your research so you can make an informed decision should you choose to have a C-section and to give you some healing tips in case it is a medical necessity.

Further suggestions: Read *The Essential C-Section Guide: Pain Control, Healing at Home, Getting Your Body Back, and Everything Else You Need to Know About a Cesarean Birth* by Maureen Connolly and Dana Sullivan. Check out the C-section Healing Kit from Earth Mama Angel Baby and the Postpartum Recovery Pack (www.earthmamaangelbaby.com), which address all of the unpleasantness you may experience and provide soothing comfort and pampering. Our Hot Products editor Natalie Klein insists that the Belly Bandit (www.bellybandit.com) helped her heal after her C-section and gives it her highest recommendation!

Doulas:
The Assistant Formerly Known as "Midwife"

An ancient tradition that has become a growing trend again in the United States is having a doula as a resource and support system during your pregnancy. Doulas are professionally trained and experienced women who give emotional and physical aid during pregnancy and labor. They can assist you in a home birth or as a source of support and advocate in the hospital. The doula's participation supplements the husband's role. After the baby is born, doulas also teach infant care, breastfeeding, and how to track for signs of postpartum depression. Go to www.doulas.org and www.doulanetwork.com for more information.

In your quest for information, you may want to watch Ricki Lake's eyebrow-raising documentary (www.thebusinessofbeingborn.com), which takes a look at natural home births with doulas versus hospital births. The film profiles many home births, including Ricki's own

birthing experience. On Ricki's website www.mybest
birth.com, you can watch video clips of celebrity moms
discussing their birth experiences.

At 10:27 p.m., my heart was beating vigor-
ously as I drove through one yellow light after
another. Things were definitely not going according to plan. Two years back, we were in
labor for three days before my son made his
grand entrance. Tonight, things were moving
much faster. The first contraction came just
over an hour ago at 9:00 p.m. It was a big-
gie. I suggested to my wife that she relax and
take a shower; we would see how the night
goes and decide what to do in the morning.
As she showered, I packed "the bag," notified
our doula to be on call, and put our babysitter
on alert just in case.

I was fully prepared for a long night of laboring at home. Then she came out of the shower
and told me with a serious face that she felt
like she had to push. I calmly asked her not to
and promptly helped her dress, while at the
same time calling the doula to the hospital
and getting the babysitter right over.

Twenty minutes and one ruptured "bag of
waters" later, we were at the hospital navigating our way to labor and delivery. The triage
nurse did a quick assessment and alerted us
all that the baby was crowning, after which
they pulled my wife into the closest room: a
surgical delivery suite.

In an effort to keep the room sterile, they insisted on everyone wearing scrubs. The charge nurse tossed two pairs of full body suit disposable scrubs in my direction—one for me and one for our doula. The doula slipped hers on, zipped it up, and ran in. I unfolded mine and went to stick one leg in, and when I did, the entire thing ripped apart. I am a big guy!

I pushed open the door to announce that I was coming in with no scrubs because they were too small. Someone shouted back, "They are one size fits all!" to which I replied, "Apparently not!" A resident came to diffuse the situation by bringing me a thick, pink nursing gown to slip on over my clothes. She also gave me two booties for my shoes and a cap for my head. Though I didn't understand how the nursing nightgown was going to help keep things sterile, I realized that it wasn't the right time to argue. I put on the gown and went to put on one of the booties. It didn't take long to realize that there was no way I was getting those over my size 14 extra-wide shoes. I pushed open the door again. Four minutes had elapsed since they'd all gone in there, and this time I heard someone say, "Push." "I'm coming in, the booties don't fit," I shouted. The resident insisted that I keep working on it and that I would get it.

I gave it one more go before realizing that the cap was much larger than the booties. I tried a cap on my shoe, and it fit really well.

I looked through the closet by the door and found another cap for my other shoe. Now I just needed one more cap for my head—and there were no more to be found. Once again hearing someone say, "Push," I decided to put a bootie on my head and go running in. The only trouble now was that the caps on my feet did not have treads and made the floor really slippery. I looked and felt like I was ice-skating for the first time. To add insult to injury, the bootie on my head did have tread; I had tread on my head. I walked up to my wife to try and be supportive, saying, "You're doing great, honey." She took one look at me and laughed so hard, the baby came out. Definitely not the plan we had put together.

So goes birth. No matter how much you plan, you need to be flexible when the time comes. If you can roll with the punches, you will do just fine—no matter what curves come your way.

—From Dr. Elliot Berlin,
award-winning prenatal chiropractor
in Los Angeles, specializing in
natural health for fertility,
pregnancy, and beyond

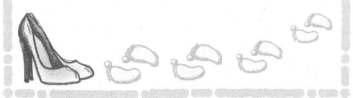

I can't say this enough: your child's birth is a very personal event. It doesn't matter how much or how little technology is involved, a successful birth results in a happy, healthy mom and newborn. So as a Hot Mom, gather as much knowledge as possible, choose your most comfortable scenario, and make the right birth plan for you. Visualize that outcome, but loosen your expectations of perfection.

The Cast and Crew

Deciding who is going to be with you while you deliver can be a challenging task, as you try to dodge hurt feelings while staying true to your vision and ideal situation. You may want your entire neighborhood—or you may be a little more private (for example, the idea of your brother-in-law filming you "down there" might be harder to stomach than a K-Fed rap). Go with whatever makes you feel at ease and comfortable; this is your baby's birth, and you should be as relaxed as possible— do not feel pressured and do not worry about hurt feelings. If you are not sure, think about all of the people who are close to you or have expressed interest in being with you and then think about all of the things you might want or need. Make sure the people in the room have a task; for example, someone might keep you calm and breathing. If your hubby is skittish, assign someone to make sure he doesn't pass out; assign someone to film, etc. Lay the groundwork ahead of time—what they can and cannot snap, at what stage they should start, and what shots you want.

What Happens in the Delivery Room Stays in the Delivery Room!

What they don't tell you in class is that you may poop, pee, or fart while you're pushing. It is part of the process sometimes, and your doctor is used to it. Don't worry or think too much about it, and if it happens to you, know that it is perfectly normal.

You never know how your body or mind is going to react at any given time until you are put in the situation. Calm, genteel women have turned into cranky lionesses, and you may yell, scream, or say things you don't mean or later feel bad about. I would issue a simple disclaimer to everyone who is going to witness the "miracle of birth": it might be laced with a few profanities or some unsightly things, and you are not responsible for what comes out (of either end!). What happens in the delivery room, stays in the delivery room!

Whatever your birth choice, be sure it is one with which you feel comfortable and confident. You can't have the best experience if you are fearful or anxious. I delivered very soon after we arrived at the hospital. The whole experience was relatively drama free. I was coherent and relaxed, and, as my mother-in-law relayed to a friend, "She delivered like she was getting a pedicure." No big deal. In a weird way, I remember feeling cheated—this was it? Seven measly pushes? I was bummed because I wouldn't have any tales to guilt my son with when he was older. "I was in labor for ninety-six hours with you . . . excruciating pain . . . see what I did for you." I'd never be able to say those words.

Movies or your favorite television shows portray the mom screaming in pain, but her hair is magically in place and makeup intact, delivering a perfect doll of a baby. Actual birth experiences, as you've probably learned in your birthing classes, can be extremely varied, but one thing is for sure: the hairdo in place and makeup intact vision of loveliness probably isn't going to hold. So, let your great Hot Mom sense of humor kick in—even if a little bit. Realizing that you can't control everything is a great step toward being a great mom.

Can't Live with Them, Can't Live without Them

Newborns attract relatives like Britney attracts the paparazzi, but the truth is you are going to need backup and lots of it! I was around children all through my growing-up years; I babysat; I was a teacher; I went to all of the Lamaze classes; I read all of the books—yet I was shocked at how much I didn't know about newborns and how much my mom taught me. What a comfort it was to have her there those first two weeks to help get me in the swing of things! Set some boundaries and time limits, but if this is your first baby, having your parents/sister/friends or whoever is willing will definitely be helpful!

Show Off!

Just as you marked your pregnancy in photographs, newborns are perfect to photograph, as they are always sleeping and angelic. You may be busy adjusting, but don't forget to schedule a professional photo shoot of the new family and of the little one. I am a firm believer that birth announcements should always have a photo, professional or not. There are many companies that will custom make your birth announcements. You can preorder many already stamped and with your address, so all you need to do is supply the photo and the info and you are all set.

Visit www.ringobaby.com, www.storkgrams.com, www.tinyprints.com, www.mygatsby.com, www.paper shouts.com, www.nestingshoppe.com, www.shutterfly. com, www.eventsininkonline.com, or www.bumper cards.com for beautiful birth announcements!

Baby Bliss and Blahs

You may fall in love with your little one at first sight, but be prepared if you don't—for some new moms, the feeling may take awhile. Lack of sleep combined with the fact that your body is adjusting to a hormonal tidal wave and the loss of the baby inside of you make it natural to feel a little "blue" or out of sorts right after the birth. Nearly 75 percent of new moms experience the "baby blues," but don't worry, it usually goes away after a few weeks, and each month it gets better. If it doesn't get eaiser, contact your doctor; you could have postpartum depression. This affects 10 to 20 percent of new moms. Brooke Shield's brave book *Down Came the Rain* really brought the symptoms of postpartum depression into the spotlight. If you feel this has a hold on you, talk to your loved ones and doctor. They will get you the help and resources you need to overcome it.

I didn't feel sad, per se, so much as numb, emotionless. I was diligent about making sure my son had all of his needs met, but I wasn't feeling that connection. I was a robot or a walking zombie, and this made me feel guilty and confused—why wasn't I feeling baby bliss? It wasn't until a few weeks that—out of nowhere—something clicked inside me. I still remember feeding him on the couch, looking into those little eyes, and it just hit me—this wave of intense love. I was awestruck and have been ever since. I haven't told anyone that before, but I am telling you—so if the afterbirth discomfort and the emotional stress have you a bit unraveled, be patient. The connection will come, it will get easier and easier, and you will feel more and more bonded. Relax and trust that.

Expect the Unexpected

Just as your birth might have gone differently from what you had envisioned, your children may be different from what you imagined them to be. They will continually surprise you.

My friend was extremely neat and sanitary—you know, one of those moms who washes everything a hundred times and has Handi Wipes at the ready for everything. She couldn't have been more organized and efficient, even through pregnancy. Ironically, out of all the babies in our playgroup, her son was the one who would find the absolutely most disgusting thing—no matter where we were—and put it in his mouth. She fished out a constant stream of small objects—a cherry stem, prechewed gum from the mall floor, and lots of strange shiny things. She even walked in on him licking the windowsill. One day we were in my kitchen after a playdate and she noticed him chomping away on a crusty piece of something. At first she thought it was dog food, but I soon recognized it as a leftover piece of meat from my pasta sauce. (This kid was good—even our dogs had missed it!) I didn't have the heart to tell her it was from last week's dinner. . . . Some of the things we witnessed coming out of his mouth made even a laid-back, ten-second-rule-abiding mom like myself shudder. How is it that her son was the one with the oral fixation? Was he rebelling already? She reasoned that, as difficult as it was for her, it was good for her—he was slowly teaching her to relax.

Growing up "little Jess," I thought for sure that my child would also be a small peanut of a kid like I was.

Was I ever wrong! My son was born big and solid and has not slowed down since. He is in fourth grade now, and his head comes above my shoulders. He was the biggest baby in the playgroup and one of the biggest boys in his class. Often when people meet us and find out how old he is, the first thing they ask me is, "Is his dad tall?" In fact, his dad isn't tall at all. It is a mystery to both of us, and to our families, and often the topic of conversation.

My point is, my son—as much as he is part of me and his dad—is his own person with his own traits. As much as we think we can predict what our children will look like or be like, you just never know.

Mom Wasn't So Crazy After All

Mothers relate to other mothers, and as your pregnancy progresses, you will slowly be accepted by the moms of the world. You will also start to see the other moms in a new light. In particular, you may slowly gain insight into, and a newfound appreciation for, your own mother. Whether you were already the best of friends or haven't spoken in several years, your relationship will inevitably change. Having a child of your own will bond you to your mom in ways that you never imagined. And as your child grows, you will understand why she did the things she did or said the things she said, why she worried so much or why she is so attached to you and invested in your life choices. If you lost your mother, you will ache for her to be with you, and she will be there in spirit.

Now, you may plan to become just like your mom—or you may strive to be the opposite. The great thing is that you get to decide the type of mother you want to be. There are so many different ways to parent and indeed so many different ways to be a good parent. The key is trusting your instincts, knowing your child, and letting his or her personality and spirit soar. As you embark on this new stage of life with your little companion, *remember that her or his happiness is a reflection of your own*. So be kind to yourself and remember, you can only be the best mom when you are the best YOU.

Before this pregnancy journey ends, give yourself credit for making it the best possible experience. You've lived through a deluge of information. You've survived the old wives' rules and "good advice." You've created a space for your baby and your spouse and rearranged your home. And you've taken care of your body and mind. Pretty amazing in such a short span of time. So while you're waiting, why not write down in your journal how this transformation can carry you into the next episode of your life—going from Hot Mom-to-be to a Hot Mom!

JOURNAL—MONTH NINE

1. What is your ideal birth plan?

_____

_____

_____

_____

_____

_____

_____

_____

_____

_____

_____

_____

_____

_____

_____

_____

_____

_____

_____

2. What was your birth experience like? (Don't forget to come back to fill this out. You will be happy you took those few minutes.)

_____

_____

_____

_____

_____

_____

_____

_____

_____

_____

_____

_____

_____

_____

_____

_____

_____

_____

_____

3. What do you imagine your baby will look and be like?

_____
_____
_____
_____
_____
_____
_____
_____
_____
_____
_____
_____
_____
_____
_____
_____
_____
_____
_____
_____
_____
_____

4. What kind of mother do you want to be?

5. For fun, write down a few things that your mom said that you think you will never say as a mom.

_____

_____

_____

_____

_____

_____

_____

_____

_____

_____

_____

_____

_____

_____

_____

_____

_____

_____

_____

_____

Baby on a Budget

Hot Moms Club Exclusive Discount Directory

Enjoy thousands of dollars' worth of discounts redeemable online only, at over a hundred of my favorite product companies.

—Unless stated otherwise, the discount code at checkout is: HMCWOMB

—Eco-Minded Mama: all companies marked with a * are eco-friendly

These are the discounts at the time of publication, websites and companies may change at any time.

Diaper Bags

Kemby: The Sidekick Baby Bag/ Baby Carrier www.kemby.com (30% off full-priced items)
Maeleebaby www.maeleebaby.com (25%)
Fleurville www.fleurville.com (20%)
Tinky Bebe! www.tinkybebe.com (10%, code: Hot Moms)

Baby and Mom Gear Boutiques

Toot Skooters LLC www.tootskooters.com (30%)
Kushies Baby www.kushiesonline.com (20%)
Mom 4 Life www.mom4life.com (10%)
Posh Tots www.poshtots.com (15% off any order over $100)

Baby Apparel and Accessories

Trendy Tadpole www.thetrendytadpole.com (50%)
Monkey-Toes www.monkey-toes.com (30%)
Bonjour Bambino www.bonjourbambino.com (30%)
Bellaziza hair clips www.bellaziza.com (30% off 6 pair, code:
    HMCWOMB or 10% off anything, code: HMCVIP)
Bonn Bonn Baby www.bonnbonnbaby.com (30%)
Ladybugs and Lullabies www.ladybugsandlullabies.com
    (30%)
*Kicky Pants www.innovative-baby.com (30%)
Minkee Tees & Calibama Rags www.minkeetees.com (30%)
*Trendy Twin Shop www.trendytwinshop.com (30%)
Fat Tie www.Shop-Fat-Tie.com (30%)
Sweet Shoes www.kitsel.com (20% *except jewelry*)
babysparewear www.babysparewear.com (20%)
*ScooterBees www.scooterbees.com (20%)
*Huddy Buddy www.huddybuddy.com (15%)
*Baby Candy www.BabyCandyStore.com (15%)
Baby Emi Jewelry www.babyemijewelry.com (15%)
Francie-Pants www.francie-pants.com (15%)
Tykecoon www.tykecoon.com (10%)
Haiden Surf www.HaidenSurf.com (10%)

*Angel Dear www.angeldear.net (10%)

TickleBug Baby www.ticklebugbaby.com (10%)

Stonz Wear Incorporated www.stonzwear.com (10%)

Stride Rite www.striderite.com (10% off any pair of Natural
Motion System shoes; *not valid in stores*)

Pediped www.pediped.com (*free shipping*)

Nursery

Re:place www.replacenyc.com (33% off hourly rate)

Crib Rock www.cribrockcouture.com (30%)

Name Your Design Modern Wall Art www.NameYourDesign.com
(30%)

Goore's for Babies to Teens www.goores.com (30%, code:
HMCWOMBPI)

*The Bean's Closet www.thebeanscloset.com (30%—a Bellini
online store, with accessories, cribs, bedding, and more)

*Scandinavian Child www.scichild.com (15% on select
products from lillebaby, Svan, Anka)

*Serena and Lily www.serenaandlily.com (10%)

*Natural Mat www.goores.com (10%, code: HMCWOMBNM)

*Aden + Anais www.adenandanais.com (10%, code:
WOMBWITHAVIEW)

Strollers and Stroller Accessories

Mutsy Goore's for Babies to Teens www.goores.com
(10%, code: HMCWOMBMU)

GoGoBabyz www.gogobabyz.com (10%)

Snuggle Me'z www.snugglemez.com (30%)
Hedvig Bourbon www.hedvigbourbon.com (30%)
The Bundle www.thebundleshop.com (20%)
*Itzy Ritzy www.itzyritzy.com (20%)
ShadyBaby www.shadybaby.com (15%)
Blankyclip www.blankyclip.com (10%)
Metrotots www.metrotots.com (10%)
Protect a Bub www.protectabub.com (10%)

Maternity Clothing

*Petite Miette www.petitemiette.com (30%)
*Rockstarmoms Maternity www.rockstarmoms.com (10%)
[bump] babies INC www.bumpbabies.com (10%, code: HMC10)
BabyPlus www.babyplus.com (20%)
Digitime capsule www.digitimecapsule.com (30%)

Baby Shower Favors

Lee-lai www.myleelai.com (30%)
Fretzels by Jill www.fretzels.com (10%)

Baby Photographers

Wildflowers Photography www.wildflowersphotos.com (Southern CA, 50% off sitting fee)
Rebecca Bouck Photography www.rebeccabouck.com (50% off sitting fee, *weddings not included*)

Mom and Baby Hygiene

Mama Mio www.mamamio.com (10%, *excluding tax and shipping, cannot be combined with any other offer*)
Honeydew www.honeydewskincare.com (30% off all Honeydew bun in the oven skin care)
*kimberlyparry www.kimberlyparry.com (30%)
oopsy daisy! www.oopsydaisybb.com (20%)

Baby Safety

Safety Mate www.safetymate.com (30%)
DoctoRx Me Book www.doctormebook.com (30%)

Birth Announcements and Baby Shower Invitations

Card Stix www.cardstixcollection.com (30%)
Pulp Factory Calendars www.pulpfactorycalendars.com (30%)
Cardstore.com www.cardstore.com (20%)
*Nesting Shoppe www.nestingshoppe.com (15%)
Bumpercards www.bumpercards.com (15%)
Tiny Prints www.tinyprints.com (15%, *minimum subtotal purchase of $50*)

Hospital Essentials

The Peanut Shell www.ThePeanutShell.com (30%)
Dear Johnnies www.dearjohnnies.com (15%, *excludes shipping and monogram*)
Belly Bandit www.bellybandit.com (10%)
B.Y.O.G. (Bring Your Own Gown) www.shopbyog.com (10%)
Daniel Green Company www.danielgreen.com (10%)

Push Presents

Marnie Rocks www.marnierocks.com (30%)
ChicBLVD www.chicBuds.com (30%)
SwankyMommy www.swankymommy.com (30%)
Shari's Berries www.berries.com (20%)
Tj&Co www.tjandco.com (15%, code: HMCWOMB15)
MIJA Jewelry www.mijajewelry.com (15%, code: HMCWOMB)
Isabelle Grace Jewelry www.isabellegracejewelry.com (15%)
Bagettes Custom Photo Bags www.bagettes.com (10% off any order over $30)
Elemental Memories www.em-jewelry.com (10%)

Baby Food and Accessories

Tasty Baby www.tastybaby.com (30%)
Beansoup Aprons www.beansoupaprons.com (25%)
TREBIMBI at Goore's for Babies to Teens www.goores.com (20%, code: HMCWOMBTR)

*Green to Grow www.greentogrow.com (15%)
*OrganicKidz www.organickidz.ca (15%)
Burpie Blocker www.burpieblocker.com (10%)

Toys/Bath toys, etc . . .

The Patchwork Bear www.thepatchworkbear.com (30%)
Boon www.booninc.com (10%)
Wubbanub Infant Pacifier www.parentingconcepts.com
   (10%, code: HMC0309)
BuckleyBoo www.buckleyboo.com (20%)
Bottle Snugglers www.bottlesnugglers.com (10%)
Child to Cherish www.childtocherish.com (10%)
Kokopax www.kokopax.com (10%, code: HOTCLUB2009)

TOP PRODUCT WEBSITES

Hot Moms Club is a great website and resource for the latest and hottest products in mom and baby gear. Visit our Hot Products section at www.hotmomsclub.com.

OTHER GREAT PRODUCT SITES INCLUDE

Savvy Mommy www.savvymommy.com
Cool Mom Picks www.coolmompicks.com
Mommies with Style www.mommieswithstyle.com
EcoStiletto www.ecostiletto.com
Celebrity Baby Blog www.celebrity-babies.com
Daily Candy Kids www.dailycandy.com/kids

BUMP ON A BUDGET

Why not try to win Swag and Baby gear? Check the following sites daily and weekly for prizes and give-aways.

www.hotmomsclub.com

www.jewelsandpinstripes.com

www.iamnotobsessed.com

www.savvymommy.com

www.coolmompicks.com

www.mommieswithstyle.com

www.upscalebaby.com

www.pregnancy360.com

$TUFF TO DROOL OVER!

If you are a fortunate mom and have more baby things than even the Octomom could use, why not donate those new or gently used products? Not only will you be helping other mothers in need but it also serves as a tax deduction (and good karma). A win for everyone!

Baby2Baby (www.baby2baby.org) and Baby Buggy (www.babybuggy.org) take your new or gently used baby supplies and distribute them to needy mothers.

*If they do not service your town or state, call your local Goodwill, women's shelters, or veterans' programs for information on how to donate.

Acknowledgements

Where Credit Is Due!

Thank you doesn't feel like enough to show my gratitude and appreciation for all the people who have supported this book and the Hot Moms Club. Thank you to Rebekah Whitlock for getting the ball rolling and believing in me from the beginning. Thank you to May Chen, Amanda Bergeron, Brenda Varda, Jennifer Rider, and Megan Byrd, my amazing editors, who should be sainted—first for their patience and always cheery attitude while working on this book, and second for their speedy turnaround. Thank you to the HarperCollins team for believing in me and Hot Moms Club. A huge thank you to Claire Gerus, my super agent, for finding this series an incredible new home.

A million thanks would not be enough for Natalie Klein. Thank you for your dedication to making each baby shower special, and thank you for your attention to detail. Your devotion to the client is remarkable; you are a treasure and invaluable to the team.

A special thank you to Rebecca Matthias. You are an inspiration and a visionary, and it is a true honor to have you support and be a part of this book. To the Pea in the Pod team, especially Judie Ashworth and Carla Blizzard, thanks for being ever-diligent and pleasant to work with. Thanks to Trista Sutter, a Hot Mom in every sense of the word: you are the sweetest and best! Stefanie Wilder-Taylor, thank you, as always, for lending your humor to this book. Thank you to Joy Bergin for being my rock; Michelle Fryer for being my right-hand everything—no matter what I need, you are always up to the task; Jennie Goodwin for holding down the fort online so I could work on this book. Angie DeGrazia and Kara Chaput, how would I ever get anything done without you two? Kelly Kimble, thank you for working your magic.

A big thank you to Alex Woodard for his incredible song "Beautiful Now: The Hot Mom's Song." It is such an inspiration, showing how moms become more beautiful *after* the baby comes.

Thank you always to my supportive and loving family—Gabriel, Mom, Dad, Kim, Jeffrey, Jenn, my goddaughter, Alana, and Gabe's dad, Bryan Dattilo. How wonderful you all are is not lost on me.

And a huge thank you to all of the amazing mothers who contributed stories and quotes. Thank you to Peggy Dattilo for inspiring several of the sections. It is a stellar collection, and I am beyond honored to spotlight all of your tips and your many experiences.

About the Author

Jessica Denay

Jessica Denay is one of the most sought-after celebrity baby shower planners in the industry. The Hot Moms Club has hosted baby showers and coordinated nurseries for Trista Sutter, Alison Sweeney, Brooke and Charlie Sheen and Ana Ortiz from *Ugly Betty*, to name a few. Jessica is the single mom of a nine-year-old boy and the founder of Hot Moms Club, one of the hottest mom groups and websites on the internet. The Hot Moms Club is on the pulse of Hollywood moms trends and celebrity baby products. In addition to contributing monthly to the Mommywood column in *Pregnancy* magazine, Jessica has appeared on hundreds of television and radio shows, including *The Today Show, Tyra Banks, CNN, The Insider, Access Hollywood,* and *Entertainment Tonight,* to name a few. She and the Hot Moms Club have been quoted and featured in dozens of national publications, including the *New York Times, USA Today, People, US Weekly, Redbook, In Touch, Life and Style, Woman's Day, Child,* and many more. For more information, visit www.hot momsclub.com or www.jessicadenay.com.

About

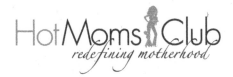

A single mom frustrated with the image of motherhood, New Jersey native and former teacher Jessica Denay created the Hot Moms Club. What first began as a fun way to boost her own confidence, as well as her friends', the group became so popular that Denay was prompted to turn the Hot Moms Club into a legitimate business in 2005. Jessica credits its success to the timeliness and popularity of their message, "You are not the best mom unless you are the best YOU!" The Hot Moms Club is an online social network that focuses on the woman as well as the parent. They define HOT as confident and empowered; it doesn't matter what age you are, what shape or size. Jessica says, "EVERY mom can be a Hot Mom! It's an attitude and a way of being." Visit www. hotmomsclub.com for more information and to join free. The Hot Moms Club also has groups on Twitter, Facebook, and MySpace.

Hot Moms Club supports these great prenatal organizations:

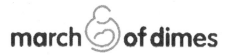

The March of Dimes carries out its mission in the name of babies, moms, and families everywhere. They are babies' staunchest advocate and moms' greatest fan and caring friend. There are millions of reasons behind their urgent mission to provide comfort and information to families with a newborn in intensive care. They support breakthrough Nobel Prize-winning research that offers solutions for babies born prematurely or with birth defects. They push for newborn screening that could save lives and prevent mental retardation, and fight for health insurance for all pregnant women and children. One day, every family will know the joy of a healthy baby. Until then, there is the March of Dimes. Visit their site at www.marchofdimes.com.

Hot Moms Club is a proud partner to March of Dimes.

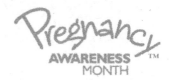

Declared and founded by holistic lifestyle expert Anna Getty, and cofounded by Alisa Donner, MSW, LCSW, May is Pregnancy Awareness Month, aka PAM. Through information, "how to" ideas, and inspiration, PAM aims to empower pregnant women and families to incorporate PAM's four key initiatives—education, exercise, nutrition & wellness, and nurture—into their life routines. PAM was created to show women and new parents how easy it can be to make healthy changes in their lives for themselves and their babies (www.pregnancyawareness month.com). Hot Moms Club is partnered with PAM, and Jessica Denay is on the advisory board.

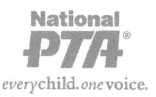

National
PTA®
*every*child.*one*voice.

Parent Teacher Association (PTA) is the largest volunteer child advocacy association in the nation. PTA reminds our country of its obligation to our children and provides parents and families with a powerful voice to speak on behalf of every child. PTA works in cooperation with many national education, health, safety, and child advocacy groups and federal agencies. The PTA collaborates on projects that benefit children and bring valuable resources to its members. (www.pta.org).

The Hot Moms Club is aligned with and supports the National PTA. Jessica Denay is their national ambassador for youth.

Printed in February 2023
by Rotomail Italia S.p.A., Vignate (MI) - Italy